Deltoid-Spring Ligament Complex and Medial Ankle Instability

Editors

GASTÓN SLULLITEL
ROXA RUIZ

FOOT AND ANKLE CLINICS

www.foot.theclinics.com

Consulting Editor
MARK S. MYERSON

June 2021 • Volume 26 • Number 2

ELSEVIER

1600 John F. Kennedy Boulevard • Suite 1800 • Philadelphia, Pennsylvania, 19103-2899

http://www.theclinics.com

FOOT AND ANKLE CLINICS Volume 26, Number 2
June 2021 ISSN 1083-7515, ISBN-978-0-323-79230-1

Editor: Lauren Boyle
Developmental Editor: Arlene B. Campos

Foot and Ankle Clinics (ISSN 1083-7515) is published quarterly by Elsevier, Inc., 360 Park Avenue South, New York, NY 10010-1710. Months of issue are March, June, September, and December. Periodicals postage paid at New York, NY, and additional mailing offices. Subscription price per year is $344.00 (US individuals), $741.00 (US institutions), $100.00 (US students), $371.00 (Canadian individuals), $778.00 (Canadian institutions), $100.00 (Canadian students), $479.00 (international individuals), $778.00 (international institutions), and $215.00 (international students). To receive student/resident rate, orders must be accompanied by name of affiliated institution, date of term, and the *signature* of program/residency coordinator on institution letterhead. Orders will be billed at individual rate until proof of status is received. Foreign air speed delivery is included in all *Clinics* subscription prices. All prices are subject to change without notice. **POSTMASTER:** Send address changes to *Foot and Ankle Clinics*, Elsevier Health Sciences Division, Subscription Customer Service, 3251 Riverport Lane, Maryland Heights, MO 63043. **Customer Service: 1-800-654-2452 (US and Canada). From outside of the United States and Canada, call 314-447-8871. Fax: 314-447-8029. E-mail: JournalsCustomerService-usa@ elsevier.com (for print support); JournalsOnlineSupport-usa@elsevier.com (for online support).**

Reprints. For copies of 100 or more, of articles in this publication, please contact the Commercial Reprints Department, Elsevier Inc., 360 Park Avenue South, New York, NY 10010-1710. Tel.: 212-633-3874; Fax: 212-633-3820; E-mail: reprints@elsevier.com.

Contributors

CONSULTING EDITOR

MARK S. MYERSON, MD
Visiting Professor of Orthopedic Surgery, University of Colorado, Past President American Orthopedic Foot and Ankle Society, Consulting Editor, Foot and Ankle Clinics of N. America, Executive Director and Founder, Steps2Walk, Colorado, USA

EDITORS

GASTÓN SLULLITEL, MD
Orthopaedics, Foot and Ankle Surgery Department, J Slullitel Institute of Orthopaedics, Rosario, Santa Fe, Argentina

ROXA RUIZ, MD
Senior Attending Surgeon, Center of Excellence for Foot and Ankle Surgery, Kantonsspital Baselland, Liestal, Switzerland

AUTHORS

ALEXEJ BARG, MD
Professor and Head of Foot and Ankle Surgery, Department of Orthopaedics, Trauma and Reconstructive Surgery, University of Hamburg, Hamburg, Germany; Adjunct Full Professor, Department of Orthopaedics, University of Utah, Salt Lake City, Utah, USA

DANIEL BAUMFELD, MD, PhD
Adjunct Professor, Department of Locomotor Apparatus, Federal University of Minas Gerais, UFMG, Brazil

JARRETT D. CAIN, DPM, MSc
Associate Professor, Department of Orthopaedic Surgery, University of Pittsburgh School of Medicine, University of Pittsburgh Physicians, Pittsburgh, Pennsylvania, USA

JUAN PABLO CALVI, MD
Foot and Ankle Surgery Department, J Slullitel Institute of Orthopaedics, Rosario, Santa Fe, Argentina

MIKI DALMAU-PASTOR, PhD
Human Anatomy Unit, Department of Pathology and Experimental Therapeutics, School of Medicine and Health Sciences, University of Barcelona, Barcelona, Spain; MIFAS By GRECMIP (Minimally Invasive Foot and Ankle Society), Merignac, France

CESAR DE CESAR NETTO, MD, PhD
Assistant Professor, Foot and Ankle Services, Department of Orthopedics and Rehabilitation, University of Iowa, Carver College of Medicine, Iowa City, Iowa, USA

NORMAN ESPINOSA, MD
Institute for Foot and Ankle Reconstruction, Zurich, Switzerland

JOHN E. FEMINO, MD
Clinical Professor, Foot and Ankle Services, Department of Orthopedics and
Rehabilitation, University of Iowa, Carver College of Medicine, Iowa City, Iowa, USA

MATTEO GUELFI, MD
Casa di Cura Villa Montallegro, Genoa, Italy; Department of Orthopaedic Surgery "Gruppo
Policlinico di Monza," Clinica Salus, Alessandria, Italy; Human Anatomy and Embryology
Unit, Department of Morphological Sciences, Universitat Autònoma de Barcelona,
Barcelona, Spain

BEAT HINTERMANN, MD
Associate Professor and Chairman, Center of Excellence for Foot and Ankle Surgery,
Kantonsspital Baselland, Liestal, Switzerland

GEORG KLAMMER, MD
Institute for Foot and Ankle Reconstruction, Zurich, Switzerland

CAIO NERY, MD, PhD
Associate Professor, Orthopedic and Traumatology Department, Federal University of
São Paulo, Brazil; Foot and Ankle Clinic

ROXA RUIZ, MD
Senior Attending Surgeon, Center of Excellence for Foot and Ankle Surgery,
Kantonsspital Baselland, Liestal, Switzerland

GASTÓN SLULLITEL, MD
Orthopaedics, Foot and Ankle Surgery Department, J Slullitel Institute of Orthopaedics,
Rosario, Santa Fe, Argentina

YANTARAT SRIPANICH, MD
Research Fellow, Department of Orthopaedics, University of Utah, Salt Lake City, Utah,
USA; Attending Surgeon, Department of Orthopaedics, Phramongkutklao Hospital and
College of Medicine, Bangkok, Thailand

SJOERD A. STUFKENS, MD, PhD
Orthopaedic Surgeon, Amsterdam University Medical Centers, Amsterdam, the
Netherlands

JORDI VEGA, MD
Human Anatomy and Embryology Unit, Department of Pathology and Experimental
Therapeutics, University of Barcelona, Foot and Ankle Unit, Orthopedic Department,
iMove Tres Torres, Barcelona, Spain; MIFAS (Minimally Invasive Foot and Ankle Society)
by GRECMIP (Groupe de Recherche et d'Étude en Chirurgie Mini-Invasive du Pied),
Merignac, France

EMILIO WAGNER, MD
Staff Foot and Ankle Surgeon, Associate Professor, Universidad del Desarrollo, Clinica
Alemana de Santiago, Santiago, Chile

PABLO WAGNER, MD
Staff Foot and Ankle Surgeon, Associate Professor, Universidad del Desarrollo, Clinica
Alemana de Santiago, Santiago, Chile

JAN JOOST I. WIEGERINCK, MD, PhD
Orthopaedic Surgeon, Bergman Clinics, Rijswijk, the Netherlands

Editorial Advisory Board

Contents

A thorough knowledge of the anatomy of the deltoid and spring ligament complex is important for treatment of deformities that impact the foot and ankle. Both ligaments are interconnected, and the study of their anatomic characteristics is better performed together than in isolation. The deltoid ligament is a group of ligaments that derives its origin from the medial malleolus, and the spring ligament complex consist of a group of ligaments that connects the navicular and the sustentaculum tali of the calcaneus. They both play an important role in stabilization of the medial ankle and medial column of the foot.

The deltoid and spring ligaments are the primary restraints against pronation and valgus deformity of the foot, and in preserving the medial arch. The posterior tibial tendon has a secondary role in plantar arch maintenance, and its biomechanical stress increases considerably when other tissues fail. A thorough understanding of the anatomy and biomechanics of the deltoid-spring ligament is crucial for successful reconstruction of the tibiocalcanealnavicular ligament, hence, to restore ankle and medial peritalar stability. Although effective in correcting the deformity, tibionavicular tenodesis might be critical, as it blocks physiologic pronation of the hindfoot, which may result in dysfunction and pain.

Undiagnosed medial ankle instability can be a prerequisite for pathogenic progression in the foot, particularly for adult acquired flatfoot deformity. With the complex anatomy in this region, and the limitations of each individual investigational method, accurately identifying peritalar instability remains a serious challenge to clinicians. Performing a thorough clinical examination aided by evaluation with advanced imaging can improve the threshold of detection for this condition and allow early proper treatment to prevent further manifestations of the instability.

Whereas tenderness, ecchymosis, and swelling over the deltoid ligament have relatively poor sensitivity, resulting valgus and pronation deformity that is seen to disappear when the patient is asked to activate the posterior tibial muscle or to go in tiptoe position is the hallmark for the presence of medial ankle instability. A pain on palpation at anteromedial edge of the ankle confirms the diagnosis. Various stress tests permit to confirm and specify the injury pattern. A pseudo hallux rigidus is the consequence of a hyperactivity of flexor hallucis longus muscle to protect the foot against the valgus and pronation deformity.

An increased interest in ankle instability has led to description of new concepts such as ankle microinstability or rotational ankle instability and the development of new arthroscopic techniques treating ankle instability. Ankle instability is constantly associated to intraarticular pathologies that contribute to generate pain and dysfunction. Arthroscopy plays an important role in identifying and treating all intraarticular abnormalities including ligament injuries. Despite a few studies are available in literature on arthroscopic treatment of medial collateral ligament injury, an arthroscopic all-inside repair of lateral and medial ankle ligaments has been proposed showing promising clinical results.

Although far less common than lateral ankle injuries, medial ankle sprains have been reported to result in significantly greater time lost and long-term disability when not diagnosed and treated accurately. Adequate diagnosis is paramount and the most important aspect is to determine whether the lesion is stable or unstable. Evidence confronting surgical versus conservative treatment in acute deltoid ligament lesions is largely anchored in the setting of ankle fractures. Ultimately treatment decisions rely on the clinical and imaging appraisal of each individual patient. This article discusses the isolated acute deltoid ligament impairment.

Chronic deltoid instability (CDI), or medial ankle instability, can happen following traumas of the foot and ankle, predominantly rotational injuries. CDI is frequently underdiagnosed or misdiagnosed. Long-term residual instability can lead to ankle posttraumatic arthritis. Adequate assessment of patients with suspected CDI is paramount. Conservative treatment can be tried for stable or mildly unstable cases, but surgical treatment is usually needed for the more severely unstable patients, or when conservative measures fail. Few reconstruction techniques have been proposed in the setting of posttraumatic CDI. This article describes our preferred technique for reconstruction of the deep components of the deltoid ligament.

The spring ligament is the main static supporter of the medial longitudinal arch. Identifying every detail of the pathophysiology of each condition in which these structures are involved is the key to an appropriate approach and treatment. Isolated reconstruction of the posterior tibial tendon present long-term results with a high failure rate. It is important to diagnose spring ligament injuries because of the probable consequences if not treated, such as acquired flatfoot deformity and loss of correction of treated flatfoot. The option of surgical treatment is discussed in this article.

The most common injury mechanism for ankle fractures with concomitant deltoid ligament injury is a supination external rotation type 4 trauma. In the acute setting, malalignment, ecchymosis, and profound edema of the affected ankle can be found. Clinical examination is a poor indicator for deltoid ligament injury. There is a lack of high-quality studies with suturing the deltoid as the primary question. The authors found 4 comparative studies that found it unnecessary to explore and to reconstruct the deltoid ligament and 4 comparative studies that find it unnecessary to explore and to reconstruct the deltoid ligament.

Flatfoot deformity consists of a loss of medial arch, hindfoot valgus, and forefoot abduction. Historically considered a posterior tendon insufficiency, multiple ligament damage and subsequent incompetence explain the different clinical presentations with varying degrees of deformity. When surgery is deemed necessary, depending on the apex of the deformity, skeletal and soft tissue procedures are considered to keep motion and restore function. Osteotomies are considered at every level where an apex of deformity is found. The recently designated tibiocalcaneonavicular ligament comprises the older superficial and deep deltoid and spring ligaments; its repair or reconstruction should be considered in most flatfoot cases.

This article deals with the treatment of a chronically failed deltoid ligament complex in the valgus misaligned ankle. This is a challenging task in every orthopedic foot and ankle surgery. Before embarking on any surgery that relates to the deltoid ligament complex, it is mandatory to analyze any underlying cause that could promote the impairment. Once this is done, it might be of value in considering anatomic reconstructions. The article provides an anatomic reconstruction technique, which should help address the problem.

FOOT AND ANKLE CLINICS

RELATED SERIES

Clinics in Sports Medicine
Orthopedic Clinics
Physical Medicine and Rehabilitation Clinics

THE CLINICS ARE NOW AVAILABLE ONLINE!
Access your subscription at:
www.theclinics.com

Preface

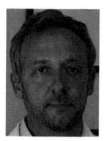

Gastón Slullitel, MD
Editor

Deltoid-spring ligament complex injuries are probably one of the most complex ankle and foot injuries. In recent years, we have observed a remarkable evolution in anatomic, diagnostic, and therapeutic concepts.

These changes were of such magnitude that they imposed the need to summarize clear and current concepts in the management of these injuries.

That is why, together with my friend Roxa Ruiz, who has a deep interest and experience in this type of injuries, we decided to publish this issue, which we hope will serve as a guide for all foot and ankle surgeons.

I want to thank our fantastic group of experts who contributed to this project. I also want to acknowledge Dr Valeria Lopez and the entire Elsevier staff for their appreciated help. Finally, a special mention goes to Dr Mark Myerson for supporting this idea, for his generosity, and for his invaluable friendship.

Dr Ruiz and I hope it will be a valuable tool that will stimulate the development of new ideas.

Gastón Slullitel, MD
Orthopaedics
J Slullitel Institute of Orthopaedics
2534 San Luis Street
Rosario, Santa Fe 2132, Argentina

Av Fuerza Aerea 2350
Rosario
Santa Fe 2132, Argentina

E-mail address:
gastonslullitel@icloud.com

Foot Ankle Clin N Am 26 (2021) xi
https://doi.org/10.1016/j.fcl.2021.03.012
1083-7515/21/© 2021 Published by Elsevier Inc.

Preface

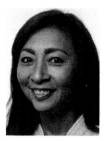

Roxa Ruiz, MD
Editor

Though progress has been made in understanding the functional anatomy and biomechanics of the deltoid-spring ligament complex, there is a lack in understanding the functional interplay of the various bundles of this ligament complex. This is particularly true when defining where motion is not physiologic anymore, and instability, with subsequent disability and progressive deformity, is present. In addition, the role of the posterior tibial tendon in the dynamic control of this functional interplay is also not fully understood yet.

Isolated injuries to the deltoid and spring ligaments are often primarily missed; thus, the orthopedic surgeon is mostly faced with the problem after onset of chronic symptoms. Meticulous recording of the history and thorough clinical investigation are therefore mandatory for diagnosis. Imaging methods may serve to further confirm the diagnosis and to reveal morphologic changes subsequent to the initial injury.

Though better understanding of medial ankle instability and subsequent biomechanical changes exist, the question remains how an injury to the ligaments of the medial ankle joint complex should be treated best.

The complex nature of these conditions makes it difficult for a single surgeon to become an expert in dealing with the multitude of pathologic conditions and using the available techniques. The authors in this issue of *Foot and Ankle Clinics of North America* are experts in dealing with the complex underlying pathologic conditions of the destabilized medial ankle joint complex and in defining adapted treatment modalities. They all provide experienced insight into the appropriate management of these challenging problems, whether common or uncommon. By sharing the know-how and experience of our colleagues, a contribution is made to understand and better treat these complex conditions.

It was a fascinating time and great experience to work together with my coeditor Dr Gastón Slullitel, and I would like to thank him especially for his tremendous efforts and patience from the beginning till the end of this project. We would like to commend the international authors on the tremendous time and effort that they put forth in preparation of their articles. Our special thanks go to Dr Myerson for his support and confidence, and everyone at Elsevier for their help in putting this issue together. We hope

Foot Ankle Clin N Am 26 (2021) xiii–xiv
https://doi.org/10.1016/j.fcl.2021.03.014
1083-7515/21/© 2021 Published by Elsevier Inc.

that our efforts will assist in the treatment of patients, leading ultimately to improved results and quality of life.

Roxa Ruiz, MD
Center of Excellence of Foot and Ankle
Kantonsspital Baselland
Orthopaedic Clinic
Rheinstrasse 26
Liestal 4410, Switzerland

E-mail address:
roxarw@yahoo.com

Editorial

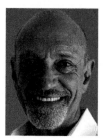

Mark Myerson, MD
Consulting Editor

I have immensely enjoyed the role as consulting editor ever since the first issue in 1996, and while I am proud of the journey that we have taken, I believe that it is now the time to hand over the leadership. I am delighted that Dr Cesar Netto has accepted this position, and I am confident that he will guide the journal with a constant level of excellence. It is hard to define what has made this journal such a success since its inception 25 years ago. We have a strong following worldwide, and it is one of the go-to sources of up-to-date information on multiple foot and ankle topics. It has been a joy to share my passion and experience by selecting outstanding surgeon leaders to be guest editors, and how we together have invited authors to present new ideas in a review format. I have learned that the only way to widely disseminate information is by encouraging and inspiring others, and this has been accomplished by bringing in international leaders as guest editors to make this journal truly global. A particular note of thanks to the editorial advisory board, Drs Federico Usuelli, Shuyuan Li, Stefan Rammelt, Kent Ellington, and Jeff Seybold. The editorial staff at Elsevier has been so supportive through all the ups and downs that we have faced together. This position has been enabling, and I have been very fortunate to come into contact with and to establish new friendships through the incredibly talented guest editors and our global contributors.

Mark Myerson, MD
Executive Director, Steps2Walk
Professor of Orthopedics, University Colorado
1635 Aurora Court
Aurora, Colorado 80045, USA

E-mail address:
mark4feet@gmail.com

Foot Ankle Clin N Am 26 (2021) xv
https://doi.org/10.1016/j.fcl.2021.03.013
1083-7515/21/© 2021 Published by Elsevier Inc.

foot.theclinics.com

Anatomy of the Deltoid-Spring Ligament Complex

Jarrett D. Cain, DPM, MSc[a], Miki Dalmau-Pastor, PhD[b,c],*

KEYWORDS

- Ankle anatomy • Ankle ligaments • Deltoid ligament • Medial collateral ligament
- Spring ligament

KEY POINTS

- The Deltoid-Spring Ligament complex plays an important role in the biomechanics of the medial longitudinal arch.
- A complete understanding of the static ligament complex is important when diagnosis and treating different pathologies of the foot and ankle.
- Reconstruction of the ligament complex via primary direct repair or secondary augmentation is essential for restoration of the biomechanics of the medial longitudinal arch.
- Failure to reconstruct the ligament complex can lead to undercorrection of deformity and progressive of the deformity.

INTRODUCTION

The spring and deltoid ligaments play an important role in stabilization of the medial ankle as well as the medial column of the foot. It is important to understand the anatomic structures in the treatment and management of more common disorders, such as adult acquired flatfoot disorder, ligament tears, and ankle sprains. Early studies of anatomic descriptions were varied[1–3]; however, a greater understanding of the pathologic mechanics has led to improved management of their injuries of the deltoid-spring ligament complex.

The ligament complex is important in multiple functions on the medial longitudinal arch as a primary medial stabilizer of the foot and ankle, the ligament complex is provided restraint against eversion tilting along with anterior and lateral translation of the talus.[4] The stability provided by the ligament complex is important with regard to the medial longitudinal arch during the gait cycle. Tear of the deltoid ligament takes place

[a] Department of Orthopaedic Surgery, University of Pittsburgh School of Medicine, University of Pittsburgh Physicians, Pittsburgh, PA, USA; [b] Human Anatomy Unit, Department of Pathology and Experimental Therapeutics, School of Medicine and Health Sciences, University of Barcelona, Barcelona, Spain; [c] MIFAS By GRECMIP (Minimally Invasive Foot and Ankle Society), Merignac, France
* Corresponding author.
E-mail address: mikeldalmau@ub.edu

Foot Ankle Clin N Am 26 (2021) 237–247
https://doi.org/10.1016/j.fcl.2021.03.001

when increased foot eversion takes place and this has shown to account for 10% to 15% of ankle sprains.[5]

ANATOMY
Deltoid Ligament

The deltoid ligament is a group of ligaments that derives its origin from the medial malleolus, where 2 colliculi (1 anterior and 1 posterior) can be found, separated by an intercollicular sulcus. This ligament complex has insertions at talus, calcaneus, and navicular bones, as well as into the superomedial calcaneonavicular ligament, acquiring a delta shape.[6]

Cadaveric studies reported that the deltoid ligament has multiple compositions along with variations.[7] Components of the deltoid ligament consist of superficial and deep layers and each layer of the deltoid ligament complex provides a specific supportive function to the ankle joint, and collectively to prevent lateral subluxation of the talus in severe ankle fractures.[8]

The superficial layer consist of the following ligaments: (1) tibiospring ligament, (2) tibionavicular ligament, (3) superficial tibiotalar, and (4) tibiocalcaneal ligament (**Fig. 1**).

1. Tibiospring ligament: originates from the anterior segment of the anterior colliculus and travels plantar to insert on the superior border of the superomedial calcaneonavicular ligament.[9] This ligament has also been described as tibioligamentous fascicle.
2. Tibionavicular ligament: originates from the anterior border of the anterior colliculus and extends to the dorso medial corner of the anterior margin of the navicular, making it the most anterior aspect of the superficial deltoid ligaments.[10]
3. Superficial tibiotalar: originates from the posterior-medial part of the anterior colliculus and the medial surface of the posterior colliculus and inserts on the posteromedial talus.[11]

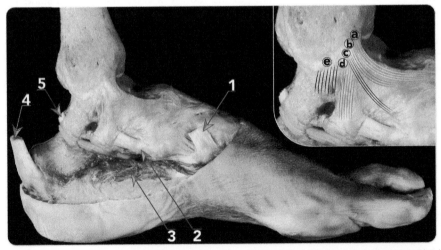

Fig. 1. Medial view of an osteo-articular dissection of the deltoid ligament. 1. Anterior tibial tendon. 2. Posterior tibial tendon. 3. Abductor hallucis muscle. 4. Calcaneal tendon. 5. Flexor hallucis longus tendon. Upper right corner: magnified view of the deltoid ligament and its fascicles. (a) Tibionavicular fascicle. (b) Anterior tibiotalar fascicle (Deep layer). (c) Tibiospring fascicle. (d) Tibiocalcaneal fascicle. (e) Posterior tibiotalar fascicle.

4. Tibiocalcaneal ligament: originates from the medial aspect of the anterior colliculus of the medial malleolus and inserts on the medial border of the sustentaculum tali of the talus and the superomedial calcaneonavicular ligament.[12]

The nomenclature of the superficial ligaments has varied but there has been increased consensus that the tibiospring and tibionavicular ligaments are consistently present while the tibiotalar and tibiocalcaneal ligaments differ in their presence in the deltoid ligament complex.[6,13] The superficial ligaments provide resistance against valgus and external rotation of talus in the tibiotalar joint.[14] Although the superficial layer is separated from the deep layer by adipose tissue, the posterior and middle portion of the ligaments has a strong attachment to the tendon sheath of the posterior tibial tendon sheath.[15]

The deep layer consists of the following ligaments:

1. Posterior tibiotalar ligament: originates from the intercollicular sulcus, the entire anterior surface of the posterior colliculus, and the upper segment of the posterior surface of the anterior colliculus. The fibers divide into 2 bands with an intra-articular one reaching the posteromedial tubercle of the talus and an extrasynovial one inserting into the talus posteriorly.[16]
2. Anterior tibiotalar ligament: originates from the tip of the anterior colliculus and the anterior part of the intercollicular groove and inserts on the medial surface of the talus distal to the anterior segment of the comma-shaped talar articular surface[17]

The deep layer of the deltoid complex provides stabilization to the ankle joint against plantarflexion by preventing lateral displacement of the talus along with restraint against external rotation of the talus.[18]

Previous cadaveric studies have become more consistent in their description of the deltoid anatomic complex. Boss and Hintermann[19] found that the tibiocalcaneal and tibiospring ligaments were the longest bands, and the tibiocalcaneal and posterior deep tibiotalar ligaments were the thickest. However, Siegler and colleagues[20] and Panchani and colleagues[21] both found the talonavicular ligament to be the longest bands of the deltoid complex and the deep posterior tibiotalar ligament to be thickest in the latter study only. Panchani and colleagues[21] also found variants in the deep ligament band located between the anterior tibiotalar ligament and posterior tibiotalar ligament and a ligament part of the superficial layer attached directly posterior to the sustentaculum tali on the medial surface of the calcaneus.

Haynes and colleagues[22] found the arterial blood supply to the deltoid complex to consist of 3 separate extraosseous sources from the medial tarsal, anterior tibial, and posterior tibial arteries. In addition, 2 intraosseous sources of vascular supply exist: from the ligament origin at the medial malleolus and at its insertion on the medial aspect of the talus.

As an essential static stabilizer of the medial ankle joint stabilizer, an injury to the deltoid complex can lead to displacement of the talus or tilt it within the ankle mortise.[23] Within the deltoid complex, the superficial layers provide resistance against external rotation and valgus stress of the ankle and hindfoot, whereas the deep layer resists against ankle eversion and lateral migration of the talus.[24] This is important during the gait cycle, as any injury to the deltoid complex affects not only the medial longitudinal arch but tibial rotation and foot inversion-eversion.[25–27]

Spring Ligament Complex

The Spring Ligament Complex consists of a group of ligaments that connect the navicular and the sustentaculum tali of the calcaneus. Its primary role is to support the head of the talus and the articular surface of the talonavicular joint.[28] The ligament complex is covered dorsally by fibrocartilage and articulates through a small triangular surface located at the medial side of the head of the talus[29] as the structures form an acetabulum pedis formed by the navicular, the anterior, and middle calcaneal articulating surfaces. The strength of the spring ligament complex has been reported to be 477N[30] and to consist of 2 distinct ligamentous bands: the superomedial calcaneonavicular ligament and the inferomedial calcaneonavicular ligament[31] (**Fig. 2**).

1. Superomedial calcaneonavicular ligament: originates from medial and anterior borders of the sustentaculum tali to insert on the superomedial aspect of the navicular and, to a lesser degree, on the lateral aspect of the tuberosity of the navicular.[32] Other studies have shown that it inserts anteriorly on the dorsal, medial, and plantar margins of the medial third of the navicular.[31] This portion of the spring ligament connects with tibionavicular, tibiospring, and tibiocalcaneal components of the

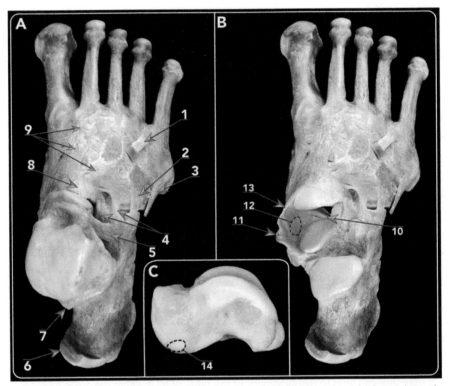

Fig. 2. Osteo-articular dissection of the spring ligament complex in a right foot where the toes have been disarticulated. (*A*) Superior view of the foot. (*B*) Superior view of the foot with the talus removed. (*C*) Medial view of a right talus. 1. Peroneus tertius tendon. 2. Dorsolateral calcaneocuboid ligament. 3. Peroneus brevis tendon. 4. Bifurcate ligament (calcaneonavicular and calcaneocuboid components). 5. Cervical ligament. 6. Calcaneal tendon. 7. Posterolateral talar tubercle. 8. Dorsal talonavicular ligament (cut). 9. Dorsal tarsal ligaments. 10. Inferior calcaneonavicular ligament. 11. Tibialis posterior tendon. 12. Fibrocartilaginous area of the superomedial calcaneonavicular ligament. 13. Superomedial calcaneonavicular ligament. 14. Articular surface of the talus for the superomedial calcaneonavicular ligament. (*From* Bastias GF, Dalmau-Pastor M, Astudillo C, et al. Spring ligament instability. Foot Ankle Clin. 2018;23(4):659-678; with permission.)

superficial deltoid ligament and is also in close relation with the posterior tibialis tendon, whereas its lateral portion articulates with the head of the talus (**Fig. 3**).

2. Inferior calcaneonavicular ligament: originates as a trapezoidal bundle of fibers from the inferior surface of the calcaneus, known as the coronoid fossa, between the anterior and medial borders of the sustentaculum tali. The trapezoidal ligament inserts on the inferior surface of the navicular to support the inferior part of the talus (**Fig. 4**).

3. Midplantar oblique ligament: Tanigushi and colleagues[33] identified a third ligament that runs independently from the other 2 ligaments inferior to the fibrocartilaginous

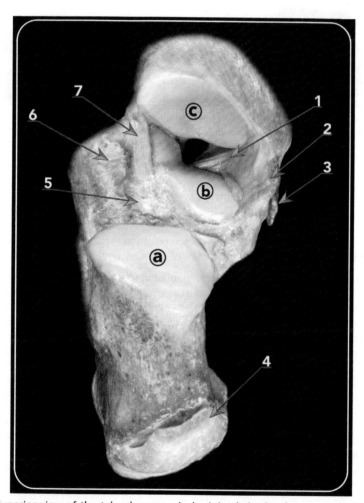

Fig. 3. Superior view of the talocalcaneonavicular joint (talus has been removed) and the Spring Ligament Complex. *a.* Posterior subtalar articular surface of the calcaneus. *b.* Anterior subtalar articular surface of the calcaneus. *c.* Posterior articular surface of the navicular. 1. Inferior calcaneonavicular ligament. 2. Superomedial calcaneonavicular ligament. 3. Tibialis posterior tendon. 4. Calcaneal tendon. 5. Interosseous talocalcaneal ligament (cut). 6. Cervical ligament (cut). 7. Calcaneonavicular component of the bifurcate ligament. (From Bastias GF, Dalmau-Pastor M, Astudillo C, et al. Spring ligament instability. Foot Ankle Clin. 2018;23(4):659-678; with permission.)

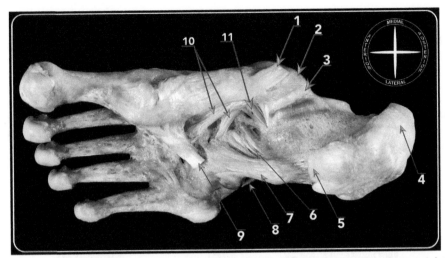

Fig. 4. Plantar view of an osteo-articular dissection of the spring ligament complex in a right foot where the toes have been disarticulated. 1. Tibialis posterior tendon. 2. Superomedial calcaneonavicular ligament. 3. Sustentaculum tali. 4. Calcaneal tendon. 5. Plantar aponeurosis. 6. Plantar calcaneocuboid ligament. 7. Long plantar ligament. 8. Peroneus brevis tendon. 9. Peroneus longus tendon. 10. Expansions of tibialis posterior tendon. 11. Inferior calcaneonavicular ligament. (From Bastias GF, Dalmau-Pastor M, Astudillo C, et al. Spring ligament instability. Foot Ankle Clin. 2018;23(4):659-678; with permission.)

surface. These fibers arise from the notch between the anterior and middle calcaneal facets and insert on the tuberosity of the navicular

Multiple descriptions have been used in relation to the anatomy of the spring ligament. Davis and colleagues[34] performed a cadaveric dissection with detailed descriptions of the gross anatomy of the superomedial calcaneonavicular ligament and inferior calcaneonavicular ligaments. The investigators found 2 definitive anatomic structures with histologic properties that suggest significant load bearing. Mousavian and colleagues[35] described that the ligament consists of 3 main bundles of the spring ligament (superomedial, inferomedial, and inferocentral) with attachments to the superficial deltoid ligament. The study by Taniguchi and colleagues[36] described a third additional component of the spring ligament complex as a midplantar oblique ligament that is distinct from the superomedial and inferior portions. Cromeens and colleagues[37] performed cadaveric studies and found the tibiospring component of the medial collateral ligament of the ankle was part of the spring ligament complex, highlighting the intimate functional relationship between both complexes.

Other anatomic findings of Davis and colleagues[34] showed the superomedial calcaneal ligament is wider, longer, and thicker, along with being more than twice as strong as the inferior calcaneal ligament, with an average load to failure of 665.5 N compared with 291.4 N, respectively.

The vascular supply of the spring ligament complex originates from the calcaneal branches of the medial plantar artery.[34] The proximal blood supply comes from the calcaneal branches of the medial plantar artery to supply by penetrating the ligament both directly and through the origin of the sustentaculum tali to supply the proximal and plantar one-third to one-half of the ligament.[34] Distally, the spring ligament complex blood supply comes from the medial plantar artery's navicular branches as it penetrates the ligament directly and through the navicular insertion to provide the vascularity for the distal and plantar one-third to one-half of the ligament complex. With the vascularity proximal and distally, an avascular area is present at the central third of the spring ligament complex.[34]

The spring ligament complex with the anterior and middle facets of the calcaneus, and the proximal portion of the navicular provides stability and support to the talar head and talonavicular joint through the midstance of gait. Moreover, is believed to provide medial longitudinal arch support and to provide kinetic coupling between he hindfoot and the forefoot.[31] Reeck and colleagues[38] demonstrated that contact forces in the calcaneonavicular ligament are much lower than in other talar articulations. Davis and colleagues[34] showed histologically that the superomedial calcaneonavicular ligament formed a fibrocartilaginous plate secondary to repetitive loads, and that the inferior calcaneal ligament presents organized longitudinal fibers to resist tensile forces.

The posterior tibial tendon is the primary dynamic stabilizer of the medial longitudinal arch. If it decreases in function, the spring and deltoid ligament stress increases, which can lead to its progressive attenuation and a decrease in the static stabilization of the medial longitudinal arch, which in turn can cause a flatfoot deformity.[39–44] Jennings and Christensen[45] determined in a cadaveric study that the spring ligament complex deficiency takes place in combination with posterior tibial tendon insufficiency in flatfoot deformity.

As part of the static soft tissue restraints of the medial longitudinal arch, the spring ligament complex often shows an injury pattern within flatfoot biomechanics. Based on MRI findings of posterior tibial tendon insufficiency, Deland and colleagues[46] found the ligament structures to be most commonly involved in acquired flatfoot deformity, with one of the most affected being the spring ligament complex. As a result of the study, 74% of patients with posterior tibial tendon insufficiency demonstrated some degree of spring ligament complex pathology on MRI evaluations.

Nevertheless, isolated injuries to the spring ligament complex can be present with a normal posterior tibial tendon. Patients commonly present with symptoms of injuries secondary to related eversion of the hindfoot. These injuries can lead to isolated symptoms of unilateral flatfoot deformity that is present in the form of valgus of the hindfoot, flattening of the arch with abduction of the forefoot oftentimes. Tryfonidis and colleagues[47] also described clinical signs of inability to perform a single leg heel rise, tiptoe standing on the affected side with partial restoration of medial arch, but with persistent forefoot abduction and heel valgus.

Whether isolated or in combination with posterior tendon pathology; the diagnosis of spring ligament complex depends on clinical examination, radiologic examination, and direct intraoperative inspection. Standard weight-bearing radiographic evaluation continues to be the initial study for evaluation of any suspicion of spring ligament complex injury, as Williams and colleagues[48] reported a significant association between an increased Meary talus-first metatarsal angle and spring ligament complex injury on MRI. MRI sensitivity of spring ligament insufficiency on MRI is reported to range from 55% to 77%, whereas specificity is 100%[49] with increased signal changes on T2-weighted sequences associated with thickening (>5 mm) or thinning (<2 mm) of the superior medial calcaneal navicular ligament.[50] Superior medical calcaneal navicular ligament has been shown to be best visualized in coronal and axial planes with a normal thickness is between 2 mm and 4 mm, whereas inferior calcaneal navicular and the midplantar oblique ligaments are best visualized in the axial plane but are also seen in sagittal and coronal images.[51] The midplantar oblique band has been shown to be the thinnest portion, with a mean thickness of 2.8 mm (1–5 mm), whereas the inferior calcaneal navicular ligament is short with a mean thickness of 4 mm (2–6 mm).[52] Intraoperative visualization of the spring ligament complex is necessary for appropriate surgical repair. The technique that provides visualization of the all portions of the spring ligament complex suggest positioning the ankle and hindfoot in inversion with plantar retraction of the posterior tibial tendon.[53]

When dealing with these injuries, the goal is to provide a stable functional foot that decreases the stress on the medial spring ligament structures across the talonavicular joint and maintains correction of the deformity. This may involve direct repair or indirect reconstruction of the spring ligament complex. Commonly this has been done as an adjunctive procedure with bone procedures such as medializing sliding calcaneal osteotomy, lateral column lengthening, and flexor digitorum longus transfer. These procedures are done in a flatfoot deformity with the hope of preventing progression to more severe rigid collapse of the midfoot. In more isolated spring ligament complex injuries, direct repair or reconstruction depending on the quality of tissue after injury can be done without adjunctive procedures.

To understand the importance of the spring ligament complex, various cadaveric studies have explored its importance in flatfoot deformity and the role it plays in reconstruction for surgical correction. Deland and colleagues[54] noted an increase on the severity of flatfoot deformity with release of the spring ligament complex and medial aspect of the calcaneocuboid joint, with the long plantar ligament.

Tan and colleagues[55] sectioned the medial ligamentous structures and capsule, including the spring ligament complex, to create a flatfoot deformity that was loaded pre and post ligament sectioning. Reconstruction of the spring ligamentous complex with split tibialis anterior tendon resulted in a significant radiographic improvement in the talus-first metatarsal angle along with an increase in the medial cuneiform height in comparison with the presurgical flatfoot model.[55] Thordarson and colleagues[56] divided the spring ligament complex along with the anteromedial subtalar joint capsule, and plantar fascia to recreate a flatfoot deformity.

Spring ligament reconstruction was performed with a portion of the peroneus longus and split tibialis anterior tendon graft; the investigators were the first to describe this technique for spring ligament reconstruction as it provided greater correction of the flatfoot deformity in the sagittal and transverse planes across all loads.[55]

Baxter and colleagues[57] combined reconstruction of the superficial deltoid ligament and superomedial spring ligament for nonanatomic ligamentous reconstruction in a cadaveric flatfoot model. As a result of their findings, greater deformity correction was obtained with an anatomic reconstruction of the spring ligament alone compared with a nonanatomic ligamentous reconstruction. These studies show the importance of reconstruction of the spring ligament complex when the native anatomic tissues show radiological and intraoperative signs of attenuation with or without degeneration that disqualify for direct repair.

SUMMARY

Understanding the anatomic structures of the deltoid and spring ligament complex is important for treatment of deformities that impact the foot and ankle. Biomechanics of the ligament complex provides stabilization against talar abduction and hindfoot eversion. Pathology of eversion mechanics impacts the ligament complex whether it is medial ankle sprain or posterior tibial tendon dysfunction.

The deltoid ligament provides stability to the medial arch by primarily limiting abduction of the talus in the ankle joint and eversion of hindfoot while the spring ligament limits the restraint of the talonavicular joint in eversion and plantarflexion.

Understanding the anatomic ligament complex allows for understanding of multiple techniques for anatomic and nonanatomic reconstruction.

DISCLOSURE

The authors have nothing to disclose.

REFERENCES

1. Federative committee on anatomical terminology. Anatomical terminology. Stuttgart: Thieme; 1998.
2. Pankovich AM, Shivaram MS. Anatomical basis of variability in injuries of the medial malleolus and the deltoid ligament I. Anatomical studies. Acta Orthop Scand 1979;50(2):217–23.
3. Rasmussen O. Stability of the ankle joint: analysis of the function and traumatology of the ankle ligaments. Acta Orthop Scand 1985;56(Suppl):1–75.
4. Michelson JD, Hamel AJ, Buczek FL, et al. The effect of ankle injury on subtalar motion. Foot Ankle Int 2004;25(9):639–46.
5. Waterman BR, Belmont PJ Jr, Cameron KL, et al. Risk factors for syndesmotic and medial ankle sprain: role of sex, sport, and level of competition. Am J Sports Med 2011;39(5):992–8.
6. Savage-Elliott I, Murawski CD, Smyth NA, et al. The deltoid ligament: an in-depth review of anatomy, function, and treatment strategies. Knee Surg Sports Traumatol Arthrosc 2013;21:1316–27.
7. Barnes DJ. Anatomy of lower extremity. Marietta, OH: CBLS; 2003.
8. Hogan MV, Dare DM, Deland JT. Is deltoid and lateral ligament reconstruction necessary in varus and valgus ankle osteoarthritis, and how should these procedures be performed? Foot Ankle Clin 2013;18(3):517–27.
9. Sarrafian's anatomy of the foot and ankle: descriptive, topographical, functional. 3rd Edition. Philadelphia: Lippincott Williams & Wilkins; 2011.
10. Campbell KJ, Michalski MP, Wilson KJ, et al. The ligament anatomy of the deltoid complex of the ankle: a qualitative and quantitative anatomical study. J Bone Joint Surg Am 2014;96(1–10):e62.
11. Pankovich AM, Shivaram MS. Anatomical basis of variability in injuries of the medial malleolus and the deltoid ligament: I. Anatomical studies. Acta Orthop Scand 1979;50:217.
12. Barclay-Smith E. The astragalo-calcaneo-navicular joint. J Anat Physiol 1896; 30:390.
13. Milner CE, Soames RW. Anatomy of the collateral ligaments of the human ankle joint. Foot Ankle Int 1998;19:757–60.
14. Beals TC, Crim J, Nickisch F. Deltoid ligament injuries in athletes: techniques of repair and reconstruction. Oper Tech Sports Med 2010;18(1):11–7.
15. Golanó P, Vega J, de Leeuw AJ, et al. Anatomy of the ankle ligaments: a pictorial essay. Knee Surg Sports Traumatol Arthrosc 2010;18:557–69.
16. Beau A. Recherches sur le développement et la constitution morphologiques de l'articulation du cou-de-pied chez l'homme. Arch Anat Histol Embryol 1939; 26:238.
17. Pankovich AM, Shivaram MS. Anatomical basis of variability in injuries of the medial malleolus and the deltoid ligament: I. Anatomical studies. Acta Orthop Scand 1979;50:217.
18. Michelson JD, Waldman B. An axially loaded model of the ankle after pronation external rotation injury. Clin Orthop Relat Res 1996;328:285–93.

19. Boss AP, Hintermann B. Anatomical study of the medial ankle ligament complex. Foot Ankle Int 2002;23(6):547–53.
20. Siegler S, Block J, Schneck CD. The mechanical characteristics of the collateral ligaments of the human ankle joint. Foot Ankle 1998;8(5):234–42.
21. Panchani PN, Chappell TM, Moore GD, et al. Anatomic study of the deltoid ligament of the ankle. Foot Ankle Int 2014;35(9):916–21.
22. Haynes JA, Gosselin M, Cusworth B, et al. The arterial anatomy of the deltoid ligament: a cadaveric study. Foot Ankle Int 2017;38(7):785–90.
23. Close JR. Some applications of the functional anatomy of the ankle joint. J Bone Joint Surg Am 1956;38-A(4):761–81.
24. Boss AP, Hintermann B. Anatomical study of the medial ankle ligament complex. Foot Ankle Int 2002;23(6):547–53.
25. Grath GB. Widening of the ankle mortise. A clinical and experimental study. Acta Chir Scand Suppl 1960;(Suppl 263):1–88.
26. Vadell AM, Peratta M. Calcaneonavicular ligament: anatomy, diagnosis, and treatment. Foot Ankle Clin 2012;17(3):437–48.
27. Golano P, Fariñas O, Sáenz I. The anatomy of the navicular and periarticular structures. Foot Ankle Clin 2004;9(1):1–23.
28. Omar H, Saini V, Wadhwa V, et al. Spring ligament complex: illustrated normal anatomy and spectrum of pathologies on 3T MR imaging. Eur J Radiol 2016; 85(11):2133–43.
29. Golano P, Fariñas O, Sáenz I. The anatomy of the navicular and periarticular structures. Foot Ankle Clin 2004;9(1):1–23.
30. Deland JT, de Asla RJ, Sung IH, et al. Posterior tibial tendon insufficiency; Which ligaments are involved? Foot Ankle Int 2005;26:427–35.
31. Bastias GF, Dalmau-Pastor M, Astudillo C, et al. Spring ligament instability. Foot Ankle Clin N Am 2018;23:659–78.
32. Volkmann R. Ein ligamentum "neglectum" pedis (lig. calcaneo n-aviculare medi-odorsale seu sustentaculonaviculare). Verh Anat Ges 1970;64:483.
33. Taniguchi A, Tanaka Y, Takakura Y, et al. Anatomy of the spring ligament. J Bone Joint Surg Am 2003;85(11):2174–8.
34. Davis WH, Sobel M, DiCarlo EF, et al. Gross, histological, and microvascular anatomy and biomechanical testing of the spring ligament complex. Foot Ankle Int 1996;17(2):95–102.
35. Mousavian A, Orapin J, Chinanuvathana A, et al. Anatomic spring ligament and posterior tibial tendon reconstruction: new concept of double bundle PTT and a novel technique for spring ligament. Arch Bone Jt Surg 2017;5(3):201–5.
36. Taniguchi A, Tanaka Y, Takakura Y, et al. Anatomy of the spring ligament. J Bone Joint Surg Am 2003;85-A(11):2174–8.
37. Cromeens BP, Kirchhoff CA, Patterson RM, et al. An attachment-based description of the medial collateral and spring ligament complexes. Foot Ankle Int 2015; 36(6):710–21.
38. Reeck J, Felten N, McCormack AP, et al. Support of the talus: a biomechanical investigation of the contributions of the talonavicular and talocalcaneal joints, and the superomedial calcaneonavicular ligament. Foot Ankle Int 1998;19(10): 674–82.
39. Sitler DF, Bell SJ. Soft tissue procedures. Foot Ankle Clin 2003;8(3):503–20.
40. Van Boerum DH, Sangeorzan BJ. Biomechanics and pathophysiology of flat foot. Foot Ankle Clin 2003;8(3):419–30.
41. Niki H, Ching RP, Kiser P, et al. The effect of posterior tibial tendon dysfunction on hindfoot kinematics. Foot Ankle Int 2001;22(4):292–300.

42. Goldner JL, Keats PK, Bassett FH, et al. Progressive talipes equinovalgus due to trauma or degeneration of the posterior tibial tendon and medial plantar ligaments. Orthop Clin North Am 1974;5(1):39–51.

43. Mann RA, Thompson FM. Rupture of the posterior tibial tendon causing flat foot. Surgical treatment. J Bone Joint Surg Am 1985;67(4):556–61.

44. Funk DA, Cass JR, Johnson KA. Acquired adult flat foot secondary to posterior tibial-tendon pathology. J Bone Joint Surg Am 1986;68(1):95–102.

45. Jennings MM, Christensen JC. The effects of sectioning the spring ligament on rearfoot stability and posterior tibial tendon efficiency. J Foot Ankle Surg 2008; 47(3):219–24.

46. Deland JT, de Asla RJ, Sung IH, et al. Posterior tibial tendon insufficiency: which ligaments are involved? Foot Ankle Int 2005;26(6):427–35.

47. Tryfonidis M, Jackson W, Mansour R, et al. Acquired adult flat foot due to isolated plantar calcaneonavicular (spring) ligament insufficiency with a normal tibialis posterior tendon. Foot Ankle Surg 2008;14(2):89–95.

48. Williams G, Widnall J, Evans P, et al. Could failure of the spring ligament complex be the driving force behind the development of the adult flatfoot deformity? J Foot Ankle Surg 2014;53(2):152–5.

49. Yao L, Gentili A, Cracchiolo A. MR imaging findings in spring ligament insufficiency. Skeletal Radiol 1999;28(5):245–50.

50. Williams G, Widnall J, Evans P, et al. MRI features most often associated with surgically proven tears of the spring ligament complex. Skeletal Radiol 2013;42(7): 969–73.

51. Rule J, Yao L, Seeger LL. Spring ligament of the ankle: normal MR anatomy. AJR Am J Roentgenol 1993;161(6):1241–4.

52. Mengiardi B, Pinto C, Zanetti M. Spring ligament complex and posterior tibial tendon: MR anatomy and findings in acquired adult flatfoot deformity. Semin Musculoskelet Radiol 2016;20(1):104–15.

53. Orr JD, Nunley JA 2nd. Isolated spring ligament failure as a cause of adultacquired flatfoot deformity. Foot Ankle Int 2013;34(6):818–23.

54. Deland JT, Arnoczky SP, Thompson FM. Adult acquired flatfoot deformity at the talonavicular joint: reconstruction of the spring ligament in an in vitro model. Foot Ankle 1992;13(6):327–32.

55. Tan GJ, Kadakia AR, Ruberte Thiele RA, et al. Novel reconstruction of a static medial ligamentous complex in a flatfoot model. Foot Ankle Int 2010;31(8): 695–700.

56. Thordarson DB, Schmotzer H, Chon J. Reconstruction with tenodesis in an adult flatfoot model. A biomechanical evaluation of four methods. J Bone Joint Surg Am 1995;77(10):1557–64.

57. Baxter JR, LaMothe JM, Walls RJ, et al. Reconstruction of the medial talonavicular joint in simulated flatfoot deformity. Foot Ankle Int 2015;36(4):424–9.

Biomechanics of Medial Ankle and Peritalar Instability

Beat Hintermann, MD*, Roxa Ruiz, MD

KEYWORDS

- Biomechanics • Anatomy • Ankle joint • Peritalar joint • Ankle instability
- Peritalar instability

KEY POINTS

- The deltoid and spring ligaments are not separate entities, but rather they form a large confluent ligament, the tibiocalcaneonavicular (TCNL) ligament; as such, they work as one functional unit, each playing its specific role.
- Besides maintaining medial ankle stability, the superficial portion of the deltoid ligament plays a significant role in maintaining rotational ankle stability.
- With loss of deep deltoid ligament, the talus progressively disconnects from the tibia and furthermore, the pivoting of the talus along the medial malleolus will be lost; this leads to a lateral shift of the center of rotation and thus a lateral shift of the articular load.
- The spring ligament plays a fundamental role in the static stability of longitudinal arch, and it also contributes to medial ankle stability.
- Reconstruction of all affected structures to restore the stability of the medial ankle joint complex may need the use of tendon grafts or/and internal braces; however, to tenodese the tibionavicular joint may be critical as it blocks physiologic pronation of the hindfoot.

INTRODUCTION

Recent anatomic studies suggest that the spring and deltoid ligaments are not separate entities, but that they rather form a large confluent ligament, the tibiocalcaneonavicular (TCNL) ligament.[1,2] As such, they work as one functional unit, with each playing its specific role. The deltoid ligament provides the main restraint against a valgus tilt and external rotation of the talus.[3–6] The superficial fascicles have been demonstrated to be the primary restraint to tibiotalar valgus angulation while the deep ligament has been shown to prevent axial rotation of the talus within the mortise.[5,7,8] Harper,[4] in contrast, claimed the deltoid ligament to be the primary restraint against pronation

Center of Excellence for Foot and Ankle Surgery, Kantonsspital Baselland, Rheinstrasse 26, CH-4410 Liestal, Switzerland
* Corresponding author.
E-mail address: beat.hintermann@ksbl.ch

Foot Ankle Clin N Am 26 (2021) 249–267
https://doi.org/10.1016/j.fcl.2021.03.002
foot.theclinics.com

of the talus, however, with the superficial and deep components equally effective in this regard.

Despite the increased knowledge of the anatomy and biomechanics of the foot, the complexity of the pathologic process that leads to medial ankle and peritalar instability has only been partially understood. It often remains unclear how specific injuries and morphologic changes of the deltoid and spring ligament complex lead to instability and deformity of the foot and ankle. The goal of this article was to elucidate the key features of the anatomy and biomechanics of the deltoid and spring ligament complex and to elaborate a rational to understand the resulting instability and deformity patterns resulting from failures of these ligament construct. This can then be used as a base for evolving treatment strategies.

ANATOMY OF THE DELTOID-SPRING LIGAMENT COMPLEX

The morphology of the deltoid and spring ligament complex has been subject to much dispute.[2]

Anatomy of the Deltoid Ligament

Currently the most accepted description agrees on 6 fascicles of variable presence which contribute to a superficial and deep component of the deltoid ligament complex **(Fig. 1)**.[9–13] The superficial portion consists of the tibionavicular (TNL), tibiospring (TSL), tibiocalcaneal (TCL), and superficial posterior tibiotalar (STTL) ligaments. The deep portion of the deltoid ligament consists of the deep anterior tibiotalar (ATTL) and deep posterior tibiotalar (PTTL) ligaments. However, controversy remains regarding what components are constant and what components are variably present.[9,12,13]

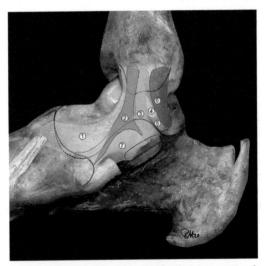

Fig. 1. Medial view of the foot and ankle. The deltoid ligament spans from the medial malleolus to the navicular, talus and calcaneus. It cannot be functionally separated from the plantar calcaneonavicular ligaments (Spring ligament). The TNL (1), TSL (2), TCL (3), and STTL (4) ligaments form the superficial deltoid; whereas, the deep ATTL (5) and the deep PTTL (6) ligaments form the deep deltoid. The TSL has a broad connection to the superomedial part of the spring ligament (SMCNL, 7), building up a sling around the talar head. The TNL is a thickening of the dorsomedial capsular of the talonavicular joint.

Anatomy of the Spring Ligament

The spring (calcaneonavicular) ligament complex is composed of the superomedial calcaneonavicular (SMCNL) and inferior calcaneonavicular (ICNL) ligaments (**Fig. 2**). The SMCNL originates from the superomedial aspect of the sustentaculum tali and the anterior edge of the anterior facet of the calcaneus.[11] It blends in with the superficial deltoid ligament, forming a larger medial ligament complex, which provides medial peritalar stability to the talonavicular, subtalar, and tibiotalar joints.[1,2] In the contact area with the talar head, the SMNCL is covered with a poorly demarcated plate of fibrocartilaginous tissue, providing a smooth transitional surface for talar head articulation. The ICNL ligament is referenced as being multifascicular; the literature is unclear as to the

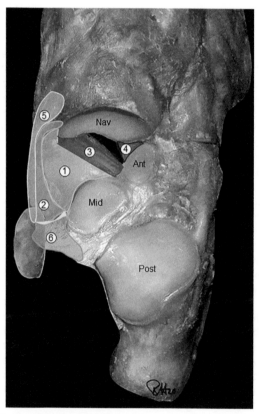

Fig. 2. Spring ligament complex, dorsal view after removal of the talus, exposing the acetabulum pedis. The spring ligament complex provides an articular surface for the talar head. Note the fibrocartilage that articulates with inferior and medial aspects of the talar head. The SMCNL (1) has a broad attachment on the anteromedial margin of the middle facet of the sustentaculum tali, coursing anteriorly, upward, and medially to the superomedial aspect of the navicular. With its triangular shape, it shares a broad insertion area with the TSL (2). The medioplantar oblique calcaneonavicular ligament (MPOCNL, 3), which is composed of 2 bundles, arises from the coronoid fossa and courses obliquely in an anteromedial direction to attach onto or just below the navicular tuberosity. The ICNL (4) also arises from the coronoid fossa to the navicular beak, being clearly separated from the MPOCNL by fat tissue. 5 = TNL, 6 = TCL, Ant = anterior calcaneal facet, Mid = middle calcaneal facet, Post = posterior calcaneal facet, Nav = navicular joint surface.

consistency of these fascicular contributions.[11,14–16] The ICNL has fibers originating in the coronoid fossa of the calcaneus and inserting on the navicular at either the navicular beak or navicular tuberosity. These fibers form 2 bands referred to as the medioplantar oblique ligament (MPOL) and inferoplantar longitudinal (IPLL) ligament.

BIOMECHANICS OF THE DELTOID AND SPRING LIGAMENTS

Although the deltoid ligament cannot be separated from the spring ligament, the biomechanics of these ligament complexes is best investigated separately to be able to understand the basic function of each one.

Biomechanics of the Deltoid Ligament

Although early studies described the posterior fibers of the deltoid ligament as being tight in dorsiflexion and the anterior fibers in plantarflexion,[17] other studies reported movements that show a more isometric pattern of elongation of the TCL compared with both the TNL and STTL.[18,19] Later, various methods were used to evaluate the biomechanics of the deltoid ligament, all of them by either separating or dissecting the bundles.[20–23] More recently, in a study on 6 cadaveric specimens, each ligamentous band of the deltoid was investigated without transection, however, with the use of force probes.[24] Data suggested that the TNL worked most effectively in plantar flexion-abduction, the TSL in abduction, the TCL in pronation (dorsiflexion-abduction) and the STTL in dorsiflexion.

The deltoid ligament was found to contribute approximately 45% of the restraint to anterior translation when no axial load was applied.[4,24,25] Harper[25] reported that posterior instability of the ankle did not increase after division of the deltoid ligament; Takao and colleagues,[24] conversely, suggested that the deltoid ligament was the primary restraint to posterior translation for the unloaded ankle.

During internal–external rotation, both the lateral ankle and deltoid ligaments were found to be responsible for restricting both directions of rotation in the unloaded ankle.[24] This suggests that rotational stability would be greatly reduced if either of the ligaments were ruptured. Stormont and colleagues[26] investigated the effect of serial sectioning of the ankle ligaments for the unloaded ankle in 3 ankle positions (plantarflexion, neutral, and dorsiflexion). For internal rotation, they found the anterior talofibular (ATFL) ligament to be the primary restraint in the plantar flexed position of the ankle and the deltoid ligament the primary restraint for the neutral and dorsiflexed position. For external rotation, the calcaneofibular (CFL) ligament was the primary restraint for all 3 ankle positions. Rasmussen and colleagues[5,7,8] studied the function of specific components of the lateral ankle and deltoid ligaments. They reported that for the lateral ligaments, the ATFL primarily restricted internal rotation, whereas combined resectioning of the CFL and posterior talofibular (PTFL) ligament resulted in an increased external rotation. For the deltoid ligament, the superficial bundles controlled both external and, together with the ATFL, internal rotation of the talus (Fig. 3). All this suggests that cooperative function of both the lateral ankle and deltoid ligaments is essential to provide internal and external rotation stability of the talus in the ankle mortise.

Hintermann and colleagues[27] and Sommer and colleagues[28] studied the role the ankle ligaments take in the coupling mechanism between the foot and the leg, especially in transferring movement between calcaneal e−/inversion and tibial rotation, in vitro. Although sectioning of the lateral ligaments did not significantly affect the tibial rotation and foot eversion-inversion for a given dorsi-plantarflexion, deltoid ligament resection highly changed the movement transfer, especially during plantarflexion.

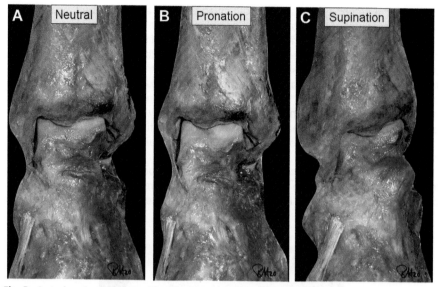

Fig. 3. Anterior view of the ankle. The lateral ankle and deltoid ligaments provide internal and external rotation stability of the talus in the ankle mortise, as seen when applying rotational forces through the tibia to the foot fixed on ground. Notice the physiologic anteroposterior shifting of talus on medial side, where no shifting is seen on lateral side. (*A*) Neutral foot position, no rotational forces applied; (*B*) pronation of the foot, internal rotation forces applied to the tibia; and (*C*) supination of the foot, external rotation forces applied to the tibia.

Apparently, the coupling mechanism of the ankle joint complex does markedly depend on the integrity of the deltoid ligament.

Earll and colleagues[3] studied the contributions of the different deltoid ligament bands to the contact characteristics of the ankle in 15 cadaveric specimens. They found that the TCL sectioning produced the greatest change in both the contact area (decreased up to 43%) and peak pressure (increased up to 30%). A similar result was reported by Siegler and colleagues.[29] These observations emphasize the role of the TCL in guiding ankle rotations on the medial side, similar to the CFL on the lateral side.

Biomechanics of the Spring Ligament

As the talus does not have direct muscle attachments, this bone has a "sandwich"-like position, which is controlled and guided by forces applied through the proximal and distal segments. Under physiologic conditions there is an equilibrium of the acting forces supported by the intrinsic stability of the tibiotalar joint. The posterior facet of the subtalar joint has a convex/concave surface like a ball-and-socket type joint. The configuration of the posterior facet allows rotational movements, which especially support accommodation during walking or running on uneven ground. The anterior facet of the subtalar joint has a flatter configuration, therefore translational movements in the subtalar joint occur more through this joint facet. The contour of the osseous structures on the lateral view is oblique, meaning that the talus has a general tendency to slide anteriorly under higher ankle loading. Subsequentially, the forces of the tibialis posterior and peroneus brevis that act distally in the functional hindfoot chain[30,31] may influence the deformity process, as both muscles cause a pulling effect, especially at the distal segment of the foot/hindfoot complex (**Fig. 4**).

In cases in which the contribution of intrinsic stability of the tibiotalar joint is missing, the subtalar joint does not seem to be able to compensate for the instability and starts to tilt, resulting in peritalar instability.[32] In some cases, the calcaneus follows the orientation of the talus; in most cases, however, the calcaneus goes in the opposite direction, resulting in a so-called "zigzag" or "z-shaped" deformity (**Fig. 5**). Such opposing movement of the calcaneus may often result in a clinically well-aligned hindfoot. However, as its height has decreased, the surrounding soft tissue structures do typically demonstrate additional loss of tension with a clinical appearance of a "floppy hindfoot."

A crucial role in the stabilization mechanism of the talocalcaneonavicular (peritalar) joint may be attributed to the spring ligament. Furthermore, the SMCNL, medioplantar oblique calcaneonavicular ligament, and ICNL create, in conjunction with the

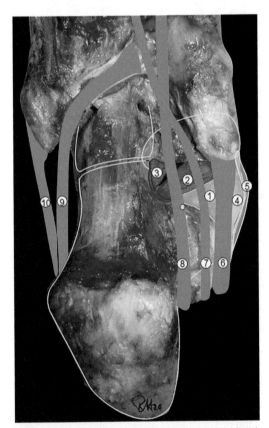

Fig. 4. Plantar view of the foot. The PT, flexor digitorum longus (FDL) ,and flexor hallucis longus (FHL) tendons run beneath the spring ligament complex, thus being active stabilizers and supporting this ligament complex. The PT muscle has the longest lever to the center of rotation of the talonavicular joint (*yellow circle*). On the lateral side, they are opposed to the peroneus brevis (PB) and peroneus longus (PL) tendons. 1 = SMCNL, 2 = medioplantar oblique calcaneonavicular ligament (MPOCNL), 3 = ICNL, 4 = TSL, 5 = TNL, 6 = PT tendon, 7 = FDL tendon, 8 = FHL tendon, 9 = PL tendon, 10 = PB tendon.

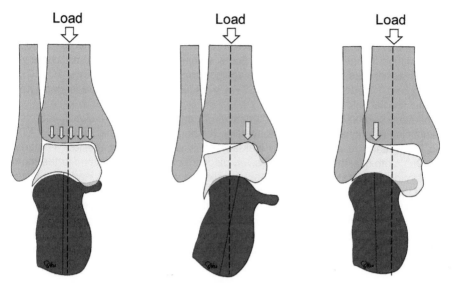

Fig. 5. Coronal view of the ankle joint complex. (*A*) When intrinsic stability is provided by the tibiotalar (ankle) joint, the talus stays when axial load is applied, resulting in a stable ankle joint complex. With loss of intrinsic stability of the tibiotalar (ankle) joint, the talus tilts into (*B*) varus or (*C*) valgus, whereas, the subtalar joint can compensate for the instability by an opposing movement. The calcaneus remains aligned, but it typically moves more toward lateral in a valgus ankle, as it does toward medially in a varus ankle. Peak joint load in a varus tilted talus is found in the medial tibiotalar joint and in a valgus tilted talus in the lateral tibiotalar joint (yellow *arrows*).

superficial deltoid (TSL and TNL), a complex of ligaments that support the talar head and thereby stabilize the medial ankle and peritalar joints. Moreover, recent studies have shown that besides preventing foot pronation, the deltoid-spring ligament complex plays a crucial role in the maintenance of the plantar arch.[33,34] Although the posterior tibial (PT) tendon dynamically supports this ligament function, it only plays a secondary role in the plantar arch maintenance, thus not being able to protect the foot against progressive flatfoot development once the ligamentous structures have failed.[35,36]

BIOMECHANICS OF MEDIAL ANKLE INSTABILITY

Besides maintaining medial ankle stability, the superficial portion of the deltoid ligament plays a significant role in maintaining rotational ankle stability. It has been shown that the loss of the TNL and TSL leads to a measurable increase in eversion/pronation without any tilting of the talus or gapping of the subtalar joint.[5,7,37,38] It has also been shown that the loss of the TNL and TSL allows an increase in internal rotation of the leg.[39] In fact, the loss of the TNL and TSL restraint unlocks the subtalar joint, allowing further eversion/pronation. It is this increase in eversion/pronation and probably also some laxity of the ATFL that may lead to symptomatic instability. Keeping this in mind, no tilting is necessary at either ankle or subtalar levels to experience functional instability.

The question, however, remains, to which extent this pronation movement is physiologic. It is obvious that the tibiotalar (ankle) joint axis and the angular configuration of talus and calcaneus in the horizontal plane are changing when the foot is moved into pronation (**Fig. 6**). Boss and colleagues[9] and Hintermann and colleagues[40] described the interval as a conjunction of a tiny layer of connective fibers between the TCL and TSL (**Figs. 7**A, B and **8**A, B). It has been suggested that these 2 ligaments get separated distinctly until the connecting fibers within the interval become tightened, thereby working as dynamic restraints against pronation force (see **Figs. 7**C, **8**C). A lesion along this interval was found in 37 (71%) of 52 patients who experienced symptomatic medial ankle instability.[41]

The deep portion of the deltoid ligament (ATTL and PTTL), plays a significant role in maintaining rotational medial ankle stability. It has been shown that loss of the ATTL and PTTL leads to a measurable increase of talus tilting while the foot is loaded (**Fig. 9**).[42] With this, the talus progressively disconnects from the tibia and furthermore, the pivoting of the talus along the medial malleolus will be lost. This leads to a lateral shift of the center of rotation and thus a lateral shift of the articular load (**Fig. 10**). These changes of biomechanics are detrimental for the integrity of the ankle joint complex and will result in progressive deformation and destabilization of the hindfoot, leading to overload of the lateral tibiotalar joint.[3] This process may become particularly critical with the loss of the PT function and subsequent chronic overload as well as degenerative disease of its tendon.

BIOMECHANICS OF MEDIAL PERITALAR INSTABILITY

The effect of spring ligament insufficiency in the development of medial peritalar instability has not been elucidated in detail. In particular, the spring ligament's contribution to the maintenance of ankle joint stability has not been investigated yet.

The spring ligament complex, particularly the SMCNL component, could be considered a primary static restraint to deformity of the talonavicular joint. This ligament is often attenuated or torn in patients with adult-acquired flatfoot deformity.[35] A large spring ligament tear leads to further progression of medial instability and deltoid dysfunction that affects the tibiotalar joint (**Fig. 11**).[34] However, it is not the only restraint, as release of this ligament does not create immediate deformity without cyclic loading. With cyclic loading, however, other ligamentous restraints are likely to attenuate, causing the development of the deformity once the primary restraint has been lost. Biomechanical models that apply cyclic loading following release of the spring ligament have produced deformities that are similar to those seen in patients with posterior tibial tendon insufficiency (PTTI).[43–45]

The importance of restoring medial peritalar stability in surgical treatment for advanced stages of acquired adult flatfoot deformity (AAFD) has been suggested.[32,46,47] However, reconstruction of both the deltoid and spring ligament, rather than isolated deltoid or spring ligament reconstruction, may provide improved peritalar stability in advanced stages of AAFD.[48]

The PT tendon has a secondary role in the plantar arch maintenance.[49] This tendon cannot support the foot arch on its own, and its biomechanical stress increases considerably when other tissues fail.[33] Both the PT tendon and spring ligament act in reducing hindfoot pronation, while the plantar fascia is the main tissue that prevents arch elongation. With increasing external rotation around the talonavicular joint, the PT tendon loses its leverage, and thus its power (see **Fig. 3**).[30,33]

CLINICAL IMPLICATIONS

The progressive kinematic changes of the talonavicular, subtalar, and tibiotalar joints can be explained by understanding the anatomy of the deltoid-spring ligament complex, which spans across and provides medial stability to those joints. The importance

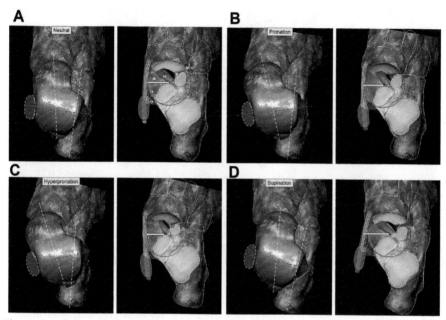

Fig. 6. Dorsal view of the coxa pedis showing the calcaneonavicular (spring) ligament complex in the various foot positions. (*A*) Neutral foot position: (*a*) The talus is sitting on top of the calcaneus with a talocalcaneal angle α of 20°. The dotted yellow line shows the position of the medial malleolus, and the dotted red line is the axis of the tibiotalar (ankle) joint. (*b*) Situs of the facets of the calcaneus and the articular surface of the navicular after removal of the talus. The spring ligament forms, in conjunction with parts of the superficial deltoid and bifurcate ligament, a strong ligamentous construct that supports and surrounds the talar head, thus providing support and stability. Note the missing bony support of the talar head on the medial side, where the spring and TSL provide the support and stabilization. As the TCL is in loose contact with the TSL through the interval, the TCL does not provide restraint against abduction of the forefoot, for example, external rotation of the talonavicular (TN) joint about its own rotational axis. The PT tendon runs beneath the SMCNL and TSL, thus having a leverage to the axis of rotation of the TN joint, which corresponds to the size of the radius of the circle given by the TN joint (*yellow double arrow*). (*B*) Foot in pronation: (*a*) The talocalcaneal angle α has increased to 30°. (*b*) The acetabulum pedis has opened medially, and the *line* of action of the PT tendon has moved laterally, thus its leverage to the center of rotation of the TN joint has decreased substantially. (*C*) Foot in hyperpronation: (*a*) The talocalcaneal angle α has increased to 35°. (*b*) The *line* of action of the PT tendon has moved further laterally, thus its leverage to the center of rotation of the TN joint has further decreased. (*D*) Foot in supination: (*a*) the talocalcaneal angle α has decreased to 10°. (*b*) The medial side of the acetabulum pedis has closed, for example, the distance between the anterior facet of the calcaneus and the tuberosity of the navicular has decreased. The direction of the medioplantar oblique calcaneonavicular ligament (MPOCNL), the SMCNL, and TSL has changed, as the navicular tuberosity has approached the medial malleolus. Note the line of action of the PT tendon with an increased leverage about the axis of rotation of TN joint when compared with the foot in pronation or hyperpronation. 1 = SMCNL, 2 = medioplantar oblique calcaneonavicular ligament (MPOCNL), 3 = ICNL, 4 = TSL, 5 = TNL, 6 = TCL, 7 = lateral calcaneonavicular ligament (LCNL), 8 = medial calcaneocuboid ligament (MCCL), 9 = PT tendon.

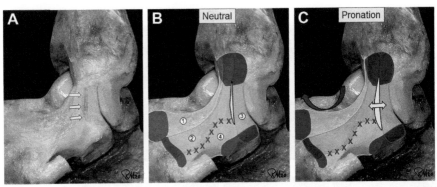

Fig. 7. Medial view of the ankle. (*A*) Ligamentous preparation showing the interval (*arrows*) between the TSL and TCL (see text). (*B*) The deltoid-spring ligament complex is shown with the insertion area of the superficial deltoid ligaments and the SMCNL (*red area*). Notice the ligamentous suspension of the SMCNL by the TSL (*X*), forming a Hammacklike construct. (*C*) When pronation is applied, the interval is gradually widened, giving rise to a dynamic adaptation of the superficial deltoid. 1 = TNL, 2 = TSL, 3 = TCL, 4 = SMCNL.

of restoring tibiotalar and peritalar stability in surgical treatment of medial ankle instability[40,41] and progressive collapsing foot deformity, for example, acquired flatfoot deformity[32,35,46,47] has been suggested. However, few data exist on the effectiveness of medial ligament stabilization methods. The reported techniques addressed damage to the deltoid[40,50–52] or the spring ligament,[53,54] often in combination with calcaneal osteotomies.[55] The independent approach may not fully restore combined tibiotalar, tibionavicular, and subtalar joint stability, as well as combined reconstruction of the deltoid and spring ligament would do.[48,55,56]

The main treatment strategy is to reconstruct all affected structures to restore the stability of the medial ankle joint complex. In the case of an extended injury with a long-standing instability, especially in the presence of a medial talar tilt, the question arises whether a primary reconstruction is feasible or whether the use of an autograft

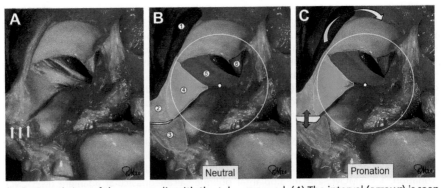

Fig. 8. Dorsal view of the coxa pedis with the talus removed. (*A*) The interval (*arrows*) is seen between the TSL and TCL. (*B*) In neutral position, the interval is closed. (*C*) When pronation forces are applied, the interval becomes widened allowing the superficial deltoid-spring ligament complex for dynamic adaptation while supporting the talar head. 1 = TNL, 2 = TSL, 3 = TCL, 4 = SMCNL, 5 = medioplantar oblique calcaneonavicular ligament (MPOCNL), 6 = ICNL.

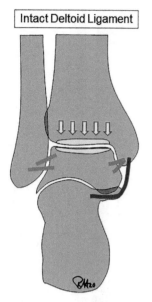
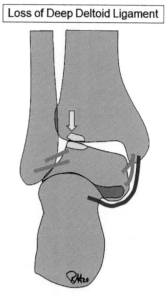

Fig. 9. Anterior view of the right ankle, showing the effect of axial loading of the ankle joint complex. (*A*) If stable, joint congruity is preserved, resulting in a symmetric load of tibiotalar joint (*yellow area*). (*B*) Loss of the deep deltoid ligament (ATTL and PTTL) leads to an increase of talus tilting while the foot is loaded, which results in an overload of lateral tibiotalar joint (*yellow area*).

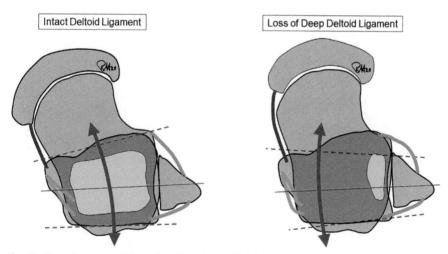

Fig. 10. Superior view of the right tibiotalar (ankle) joint; in this model, the position of talus and navicular are shown while the tibia is fixed. (*A*) While the joint load (*yellow area*) is symmetric in a stable tibiotalar joint, the talus fellows the medial malleolus during dorsi-/plantarflexion, as indicated by the *red double arrow*. (*B*) Loss of deep deltoid support results in talus tilting, leading to an overload of lateral tibiotalar joint (*yellow area*); with this, the biomechanics of tibiotalar joint changes dramatically, as the talus now pivots around the fibula (*red double arrow*) instead the medial malleolus. The talus typically shifts anteriorward when the foot starts to pronate when the foot is loaded.

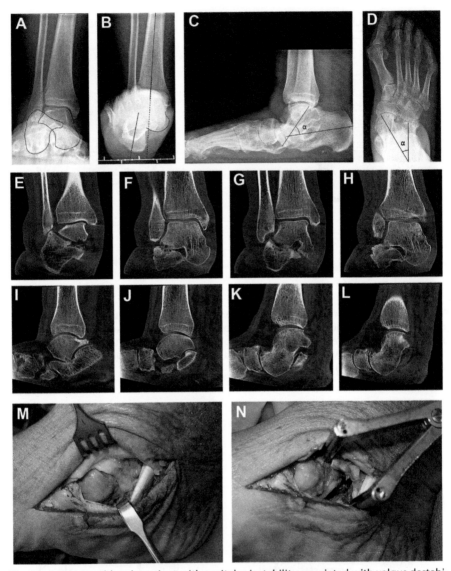

Fig. 11. A 67-year-old male patient with peritalar instability associated with valgus destabilization of the right ankle joint complex and break-down of medial arch after a pronation trauma 18 months ago. (*A–D*) Standard weight-bearing radiographs showing a distinct varus tilt of talus, a medial slide of talus on top of calcaneus with exposure of its head, a massive plantarflexion of talus, and a medial uncoverage of talar head. The talocalcaneal angle (α) is dramatically increased in the sagittal and horizontal plane. Weight-bearing computed tomography scans: (*E–H*) In the coronal plane, the talar slide toward medioplantar is seen, with subluxation at subtalar joint and sinus tarsi impingement with subsequent osteoarthritis. The medial clear space is narrowed due to lateral translational forces to the talus within the ankle mortise. Although the tibiotalar joint space is preserved posteriorly, a gapping of medial tibiotalar joint space, that is, a valgus tilt of talus, is seen in the anterior ankle joint. (*I–L*) Sagittal plane. Although the joint congruency is preserved in the lateral ankle joint, an opening of tibiotalar joint space in its anterior part is seen that gradually increases toward medially. (*M*) Surgical exposure evidences an extended tear of both the

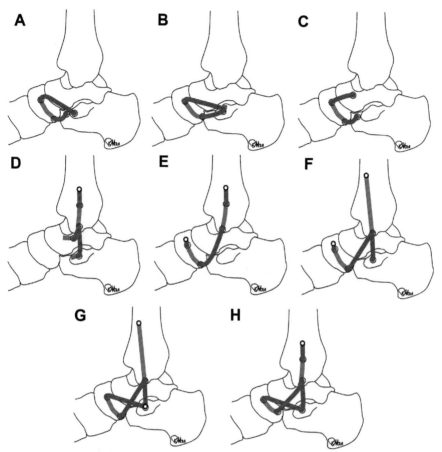

Fig. 12. Various proposed reconstruction techniques, mostly with the use of a free peroneus longus tendon graft.[48,50–55,58,62] (*A–C*) Isolated reconstruction of the spring ligament. (*D*) Isolated reconstruction of deltoid ligament. (*E–H*) Combined reconstruction of spring and deltoid ligaments (tibiocalcaneonavicular reconstruction).

or allograft is necessary.[50–52,55,57–61] Correcting osteotomies to support the reconstructed soft tissue structures may also be considered.[40,41]

A combined spring and deltoid (tibiocalcaneonavicular [TCNL]) ligament reconstruction was first described by Grunfeld and colleagues.[62] Variations in surgical technique for the isolated repair or reconstruction of the spring ligament (**Fig. 12**A–C) or deltoid ligament (see **Fig. 12**D) and the simultaneous repair or reconstruction of both the deltoid and spring ligaments (see **Fig. 12** E–H) have been reported.[56,63] MacDonald et al.,[48] using a severe flatfoot model in 10 fresh-frozen cadaveric specimens, found that combined spring and deltoid ligament reconstruction was the only reconstruction

spring and superficial deltoid ligaments, whereas the PT tendon is intact. (*N*) When distraction is applied to the subtalar joint, the amount of instability becomes obvious. Notice the spontaneous reduction of talus subsequently to the distraction.

method that significantly corrected both the subtalar and tibiotalar valgus alignment. When evaluating the lateral talo-first metatarsal angle, both the isolated spring ligament and combined deltoid-spring ligament reconstructions corrected the sagittal alignment, whereas the isolated deltoid reconstruction was unable to correct to the lateral T-1 MT angle. These findings support those of others[54,55,58] that reconstruction

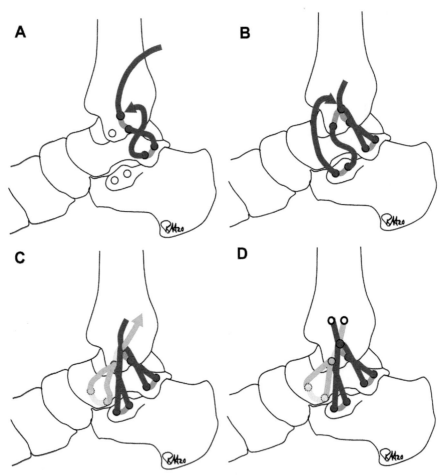

Fig. 13. The author's preferred anatomic reconstruction, using a free plantaris tendon graft that can be augmented by an internal brace. (*A*) After having drilled seven 3.5-mm holes within the insertion area of deltoid ligament at medial malleolus, posteromedial talus, and sustentaculum tali of calcaneus, a first loop is made to reconstruct the deep deltoid ligament (anterior and posterior tibiotalar ligaments). (*B*) After having tightened this loop, a second loop is made to the sustentaculum tali to reconstruct the tibiocalcaneal ligament. (*C*) A third loop (*yellow*) is done in a sling fashion to grab the spring ligament and tibiospring ligaments. Usually there is enough consistent ligament left beneath the talar head and the tibiospring ligament for a reliable fixation. If necessary, this sling can be extended to the medioplantar oblique calcaneonavicular and tibionavicular ligaments. (*D*) Final reconstruction after having fixed the ends of the graft by transosseous sutures or screws to the tibia, showing the isometric position of the 2 slings (*red*, deep deltoid and the tibiocalcaneal ligament), and the 3rd sling (*yellow*) for dynamic reconstruction of the anterior superficial deltoid and spring ligaments, thus avoiding a tibionavicular tenodesis.

of the tibionavicular limb of the deltoid ligament resulted in the best correction of talo-navicular and hindfoot valgus deformity. This suggests that reconstruction of the TNL, which spans across the tibiotalar and talonavicular joints, may provide stronger talo-navicular joint stability and hindfoot valgus correction than reconstruction of the native spring ligament alone.[64] Analogously, Kelly and colleagues,[34] using a noninvasive method of joint reaction force measurements, found an enhanced medial joint stability when additionally reconstructing the tibiocalcaneal limb for reconstruction of the TCNL compared with anatomic repair of the spring ligament alone.

However, tenodesing the tibionavicular joints is not without fear of changing the biomechanics of the hindfoot. Especially physiologic pronation of the foot in late land-ing and early stance phase, is restrained. Moreover, if it creates an acute stop of this movement, it may result in pain and disability.[65–67] As emphasized by the anatomy-based functional analysis (**Figure 6** and **7**), tendon grafts or internal braces must reroute onto the anatomic insertion area of the specific tendons on either the medial malleolus, talus, calcaneus and navicular, and they must respect the course of the lig-ament bundles they are aimed to reconstruct. This is particularly true for the TNL, which acts as the suspension of the hammocklike construct of the deltoid-spring lig-ament complex with its curved course at its superior border. Keeping this is mind, we have been using a technique to reconstruct the whole deltoid-spring ligament com-plex that avoids a tibionavicular tenodesis (**Fig. 13**). Six high-demanding athletes, one of which won a medal at the Olympic Games 3 years later, have successfully been treated.

SUMMARY

The deltoid-spring ligament complex has been clearly elucidated as the main static re-straint of the tibiotalar (ankle), talocalcaneal (subtalar) and talonavicular joint. Although progress has been made in understanding the functional anatomy and biomechanics of the deltoid-spring ligament complex, there is still a lack in understanding the func-tional interplay of the various bundles of this ligament complex. This is particularly true for defining the limit between physiologic motion and instability with subsequent disability and progressive deformity. Furthermore, the role of PT tendon in the dynamic control of this functional interplay is also not fully understood yet.[30,35,36,43]

In the past years, the use of tendon autografts and allografts have been proposed to restore adequate stability of the medial ankle joint complex.[48–55,57–62,64] Reconstruction of the TCNL, rather than isolated deltoid or spring ligament reconstruction, may provide improved peritalar stability, especially in advanced flatfoot deformity and medial ankle instability with progressive valgus talar tilt.[48] Despite showing acceptable results intra-operatively, studies are needed to examine whether they can resist against the applied forces during daily life and whether they affect the biomechanics or possibly even restrict motion over time. In any case, respecting the anatomy is crucial, in particular with the use of internal braces[56,57] and the use of arthroscopic techniques.[68]

Further studies are necessary to not only answer open questions and improve the reconstruction techniques, but also to determine the efficacy of surgical reconstruc-tion in restoring the stability of the medial ankle joint complex and overall foot function.

CLINICS CARE POINTS

- A thorough understanding of anatomy and biomechanics of medial ankle ligaments are mandatory for appropriate diagnosis making and successful treatment.

- Injuries to the deltoid-spring ligament complex might result in significant changes of biomechanics of the ankle and peritalar joints.
- Neglecting injuries to the deltoid-spring ligament complex may result in complex instability patterns that may cause deformity and secondary osteoarthritis.
- Treatment of chronic instability must aim to restore biomechanics, thus respect the anatomy of the deltoid-spring ligament complex.

DISCLOSURE

The authors declare no potential conflicts of interest with respect to the research, authorship, and/or publication of this article.

REFERENCES

1. Campbell KJ, Michalski MP, Wilson KJ, et al. The ligament anatomy of the deltoid complex of the ankle: a qualitative and quantitative anatomical study. J Bone Joint Surg Am 2014;96(8):e62.
2. Cromeens BP, Kirchhoff CA, Patterson RM, et al. An attachment-based description of the medial collateral and spring ligament complexes. Foot Ankle Int 2015; 36(6):710–21.
3. Earll M, Wayne J, Brodrick C, et al. Contribution of the deltoid ligament to ankle joint contact characteristics: a cadaver study. Foot Ankle Int 1996;17(6):317–24.
4. Harper MC. Deltoid ligament: an anatomical evaluation of function. Foot Ankle 1987;8(1):19–22.
5. Rasmussen O, Kromann-Andersen C, Boe S. Deltoid ligament. Functional analysis of the medial collateral ligamentous apparatus of the ankle joint. Acta Orthop Scand 1983;54(1):36–44.
6. Resnick RB, Jahss MH, Choueka J, et al. Deltoid ligament forces after tibialis posterior tendon rupture: effects of triple arthrodesis and calcaneal displacement osteotomies. Foot Ankle Int 1995;16(1):14–20.
7. Rasmussen O, Kromann-Andersen C. Experimental ankle injuries. Analysis of the traumatology of the ankle ligaments. Acta Orthop Scand 1983;54(3):356–62.
8. Rasmussen O. Stability of the ankle joint. Analysis of the function and traumatology of the ankle ligaments. Acta Orthop Scand Suppl 1985;211:1–75.
9. Boss AP, Hintermann B. Anatomical study of the medial ankle ligament complex. Foot Ankle Int 2002;23(6):547–53.
10. Hintermann B, Golanó P. The anatomy and function of the deltoid ligament. Tech Foot Ankle Surg 2014;13(2):67–72.
11. Kelikian AS. Sarrafian's anatomy of the foot and ankle: descriptive, topographic, funtional. 3rd edition. Philadelphia, PA: Lippincott Williams & Wilkins; 2011.
12. Milner CE, Soames RW. Anatomy of the collateral ligaments of the human ankle joint. Foot Ankle Int 1998;19(11):757–60.
13. Milner CE, Soames RW. The medial collateral ligaments of the human ankle joint: anatomical variations. Foot Ankle Int 1998;19(5):289–92.
14. Golano P, Farinas O, Saenz I. The anatomy of the navicular and periarticular structures. Foot Ankle Clin 2004;9(1):1–23.
15. Mengiardi B, Zanetti M, Schottle PB, et al. Spring ligament complex: MR imaging-anatomic correlation and findings in asymptomatic subjects. Radiology 2005; 237(1):242–9.

16. Taniguchi A, Tanaka Y, Takakura Y, et al. Anatomy of the spring ligament. J Bone Joint Surg Am 2003;85(11):2174–8.
17. Lapidus PW. Kinesiology and mechanical anatomy of the tarsal joints. Clin Orthop Relat Res 1963;30:20–36.
18. Luo ZP, Kitaoka HB, Hsu HC, et al. Physiological elongation of ligamentous complex surrounding the hindfoot joints: in vitro biomechanical study. Foot Ankle Int 1997;18(5):277–83.
19. Quiles M, Requena F, Gomez L, et al. Functional anatomy of the medial collateral ligament of the ankle joint. Foot Ankle 1983;4(2):73–82.
20. Tochigi Y, Rudert MJ, Amendola A, et al. Tensile engagement of the peri-ankle ligaments in stance phase. Foot Ankle Int 2005;26(12):1067–73.
21. Wei F, Hunley SC, Powell JW, et al. Development and validation of a computational model to study the effect of foot constraint on ankle injury due to external rotation. Ann Biomed Eng 2011;39(2):756–65.
22. Wei F, Braman JE, Weaver BT, et al. Determination of dynamic ankle ligament strains from a computational model driven by motion analysis based kinematic data. J Biomech 2011;44(15):2636–41.
23. Kjaersgaard-Andersen P, Wethelund JO, Helmig P, et al. Stabilizing effect of the tibiocalcaneal fascicle of the deltoid ligament on hindfoot joint movements: an experimental study. Foot Ankle 1989;10(1):30–5.
24. Takao M, Ozeki S, Oliva XM, et al. Strain pattern of each ligamentous band of the superficial deltoid ligament: a cadaver study. BMC Musculoskelet Disord 2020; 21(1):289.
25. Harper MC. Talar shift. The stabilizing role of the medial, lateral, and posterior ankle structures. Clin Orthop Relat Res 1990;(257):177–83.
26. Stormont DM, Morrey BF, An KN, et al. Stability of the loaded ankle. Relation between articular restraint and primary and secondary static restraints. Am J Sports Med 1985;13(5):295–300.
27. Hintermann B, Sommer C, Nigg BM. Influence of ligament transection on tibial and calcaneal rotation with loading and dorsi-plantarflexion. Foot Ankle Int 1995;16(9):567–71.
28. Sommer C, Hintermann B, Nigg BM, et al. Influence of ankle ligaments on tibial rotation: an in vitro study. Foot Ankle Int 1996;17(2):79–84.
29. Siegler S, Block J, Schneck CD. The mechanical characteristics of the collateral ligaments of the human ankle joint. Foot Ankle 1988;8(5):234–42.
30. Hintermann B. Biomechanische Aspekte der Muskel-Sehnen-Funktion [Biomechanical aspects of muscle-tendon functions]. Orthopade 1995;24(3):187–92.
31. Piazza SJ, Adamson RL, Sanders JO, et al. Changes in muscle moment arms following split tendon transfer of tibialis anterior and tibialis posterior. Gait Posture 2001;14(3):271–8.
32. Hintermann B, Knupp M, Barg A. Peritalar instability. Foot Ankle Int 2012;33(5): 450–4.
33. Cifuentes-De la Portilla C, Larrainzar-Garijo R, Bayod J. Biomechanical stress analysis of the main soft tissues associated with the development of adult acquired flatfoot deformity. Clin Biomech (Bristol, Avon) 2019;61:163–71.
34. Kelly M, Masqoodi N, Vasconcellos D, et al. Spring ligament tear decreases static stability of the ankle joint. Clin Biomech (Bristol, Avon) 2019;61:79–83.
35. Deland JT, de Asla RJ, Sung IH, et al. Posterior tibial tendon insufficiency: which ligaments are involved? Foot Ankle Int 2005;26(6):427–35.
36. Smyth NA, Aiyer AA, Kaplan JR, et al. Adult-acquired flatfoot deformity. Eur J Orthop Surg Traumatol 2017;27(4):433–9.

37. Grath GB. Widening of the ankle mortise. A clinical and experimental study. Acta Chir Scand Suppl 1960;(Suppl 263):1–88.
38. Nigg BM, Skarvan G, Frank CB, et al. Elongation and forces of ankle ligaments in a physiological range of motion. Foot Ankle 1990;11(1):30–40.
39. Hintermann B. Bandverletzung der Sprunggelenke (Teil1) [Ligament injury of the ankle joint (I)]. Sportverletz Sportschaden 1996;10(3):47.
40. Hintermann B. Medial ankle instability. Foot Ankle Clin 2003;8(4):723–38.
41. Hintermann B, Valderrabano V, Boss A, et al. Medial ankle instability: an exploratory, prospective study of fifty-two cases. Am J Sports Med 2004;32(1):183–90.
42. Close JR. Some applications of the functional anatomy of the ankle joint. J Bone Joint Surg Am 1956;38-A(4):761–81.
43. Niki H, Ching RP, Kiser P, et al. The effect of posterior tibial tendon dysfunction on hindfoot kinematics. Foot Ankle Int 2001;22(4):292–300.
44. McCormack AP, Niki H, Kiser P, et al. Two reconstructive techniques for flatfoot deformity comparing contact characteristics of the hindfoot joints. Foot Ankle Int 1998;19(7):452–61.
45. McCormack AP, Ching RP, Sangeorzan BJ. Biomechanics of procedures used in adult flatfoot deformity. Foot Ankle Clin 2001;6(1):15–23, v.
46. Colin F, Zwicky L, Barg A, et al. Peritalar instability after tibiotalar fusion for valgus unstable ankle in stage IV adult acquired flatfoot deformity: case series. Foot Ankle Int 2013;34(12):1677–82.
47. Probasco W, Haleem AM, Yu J, et al. Assessment of coronal plane subtalar joint alignment in peritalar subluxation via weight-bearing multiplanar imaging. Foot Ankle Int 2015;36(3):302–9.
48. MacDonald A, Ciufo D, Vess E, et al. Peritalar kinematics with combined deltoid-spring ligament reconstruction in simulated advanced adult acquired flatfoot deformity. Foot Ankle Int 2020. 1071100720929004.
49. Bastias GF, Dalmau-Pastor M, Astudillo C, et al. Spring ligament instability. Foot Ankle Clin 2018;23(4):659–78.
50. Deland JT, de Asla RJ, Segal A. Reconstruction of the chronically failed deltoid ligament: a new technique. Foot Ankle Int 2004;25(11):795–9.
51. Ellis SJ, Williams BR, Wagshul AD, et al. Deltoid ligament reconstruction with peroneus longus autograft in flatfoot deformity. Foot Ankle Int 2010;31(9):781–9.
52. Jeng CL, Bluman EM, Myerson MS. Minimally invasive deltoid ligament reconstruction for stage IV flatfoot deformity. Foot Ankle Int 2011;32(1):21–30.
53. Choi K, Lee S, Otis JC, et al. Anatomical reconstruction of the spring ligament using peroneus longus tendon graft. Foot Ankle Int 2003;24(5):430–6.
54. Baxter JR, LaMothe JM, Walls RJ, et al. Reconstruction of the medial talonavicular joint in simulated flatfoot deformity. Foot Ankle Int 2015;36(4):424–9.
55. Brodell JD Jr, MacDonald A, Perkins JA, et al. Deltoid-spring ligament reconstruction in adult acquired flatfoot deformity with medial peritalar instability. Foot Ankle Int 2019. 1071100719839176.
56. Nery C, Lemos A, Raduan F, et al. Combined spring and deltoid ligament repair in adult-acquired flatfoot. Foot Ankle Int 2018;39(8):903–7.
57. Acevedo J, Vora A. Anatomical reconstruction of the spring ligament complex: "internal brace" augmentation. Foot Ankle Spec 2013;6(6):441–5.
58. Haddad SL, Dedhia S, Ren Y, et al. Deltoid ligament reconstruction: a novel technique with biomechanical analysis. Foot Ankle Int 2010;31(7):639–51.
59. Jung HG, Park JT, Eom JS, et al. Reconstruction of superficial deltoid ligaments with allograft tendons in medial ankle instability: a technical report. Injury 2016; 47(3):780–3.

60. Oburu E, Myerson MS. Deltoid ligament repair in flatfoot deformity. Foot Ankle Clin 2017;22(3):503–14.
61. Xu C, Zhang MY, Lei GH, et al. Biomechanical evaluation of tenodesis reconstruction in ankle with deltoid ligament deficiency: a finite element analysis. Knee Surg Sports Traumatol Arthrosc 2012;20(9):1854–62.
62. Grunfeld R, Oh I, Flemister S, et al. Reconstruction of the deltoid-spring ligament: tibiocalcaneonavicular ligament complex. Tech Foot Ankle Surg 2016;15(1): 39–46.
63. Patel MS, Barbosa MP, Kadakia AR. Role of spring and deltoid ligament reconstruction for adult acquired flatfoot deformity. Tech Foot Ankle Surg 2017;16(3): 124–35.
64. Williams BR, Ellis SJ, Deyer TW, et al. Reconstruction of the spring ligament using a peroneus longus autograft tendon transfer. Foot Ankle Int 2010;31(7):567–77.
65. Clanton TO, Williams BT, James EW, et al. Radiographic identification of the deltoid ligament complex of the medial ankle. Am J Sports Med 2015;43(11): 2753–62.
66. Hintermann B, Knupp M, Pagenstert GI. Deltoid ligament injuries: diagnosis and management. Foot Ankle Clin 2006;11(3):625–37.
67. Vadell AM, Peratta M. Calcaneonavicular ligament: anatomy, diagnosis, and treatment. Foot Ankle Clin 2012;17(3):437–48.
68. Lui TH, Mak CYD. Arthroscopic approach to the spring (calcaneonavicular) ligament. Foot Ankle Surg 2018;24(3):242–5.

Imaging of Peritalar Instability

Yantarat Sripanich, MD[a,b], Alexej Barg, MD[a,c],*

KEYWORDS

- Peritalar instability • Posterior tibial tendon dysfunction
- Imaging of peritalar instability • Weightbearing computed tomography

KEY POINTS

- Peritalar instability has been demonstrated to be a risk factor for the progression of osteoarthritic processes.
- Multiple imaging modalities have been used to detect this condition.
- Under physiologic loading, the existing deformity does increase in most circumstances relative to non–Weightbearing conditions. Thus, a weightbearing imaging should be acquired whenever available.

INTRODUCTION

Peritalar instability describes the atypical translational and rotational motions of the talus with respect to the articulating calcaneus and talus bones that result in abnormal 3-dimensional displacement within the ankle mortise.[1,2] This specific entity may be caused by differences in articular geometry, instability patterns of associated ligaments, and applied forced to the hindfoot complex. In addition, this particular type of instability could be an important contributor to the progression of degenerative processes within the hindfoot and particularly the tibiotalar joint.[3,4] From an anatomic perspective, the talus has a unique function coupled to its distinct anatomic shape and contributes to 3 major hindfoot articulations, including the tibiotalar, talofibular, and subtalar joints.[5–10] The talus has previously been termed the "bony meniscus" due to the lack of any direct muscle attachments to the bone, and also because most of its motion is determined by forces acting from surrounding tendons and muscles inserted on adjacent structures.[11,12] In healthy individuals under physiologic

[a] Department of Orthopaedics, University of Utah, 590 Wakara Way, Salt Lake City, UT 84108, USA; [b] Department of Orthopaedics, Phramongkutklao Hospital and College of Medicine, 315 Rajavithi Road, Tung Phayathai, Ratchathewi, Bangkok 10400, Thailand; [c] Department of Orthopaedics, Trauma and Reconstructive Surgery, University of Hamburg, Martinistr. 52, Hamburg 20246, Germany
* Corresponding author. Department of Orthopaedics, Trauma and Reconstructive Surgery, University of Hamburg, Martinistr. 52, Hamburg 20246, Germany.
E-mail address: al.barg@uke.de

Foot Ankle Clin N Am 26 (2021) 269–289
https://doi.org/10.1016/j.fcl.2021.03.003

foot.theclinics.com

conditions, these acting forces are in equilibrium and are supported by the intrinsic stability of the tibiotalar joint. Conversely, in cases of an unstable tibiotalar joint, it has been demonstrated that the subtalar joint cannot fully compensate for this deficiency and begins to distort and tilt, resultantly.[1]

Numerous ligaments have been demonstrated to contribute to the stabilization of the talus within the ankle mortise.[13–17] These ligaments can be categorized into 3 groups: (1) medial ankle ligaments, (2) lateral ankle ligaments, and (3) the interosseous talocalcaneal ligament. A broad spectrum of pathology could induce instability in each of these ligament groups.[18–29] In this review article, we focus on peritalar instability secondary to the medial ligamentous insufficiency, which is commonly observed in progressive collapsing foot deformity (PCFD). The term "adult acquired flatfoot deformity" is outdated and does not adequately describe the underlying deformity.[30] In accordance with the new consensus terminology, the term PCFD should be used instead.[30]

Posterior tibial tendon dysfunction (PTTD) may lead to secondary damage of surrounding ligaments/structures, as it has been demonstrated for the spring ligament complex,[15,31–35] which is also one of the primary static stabilizers of the medial arch.[15,35] This structure runs from the sustentaculum tali of the calcaneus to the plantar aspect of the navicular bone.[15,35] Progressive PTTD may induce degeneration of the spring ligament complex with consecutive compromising of its stabilizing function, which may result in further deformity of the talonavicular joint.[30,36–42] In addition to this deformity, the interosseous ligament of the subtalar joint may also be affected resulting in subtalar subluxation, as this ligament is one of the most important stabilizers of the subtalar joint.[43–49] This combination of the pathologic plantar and medial migration of the talar head will most likely result in substantial flattening of the medial arch. It was recognized already in 1953 that the break of the medial arch can occur at different levels.[50] The ligaments supporting the naviculocuneiform and tarsometatarsal joints may also be implicated, resulting in deformities at these joints, respectively.[51–53] Consequently, as this planovalgus deformity continues to progress, the deltoid ligament subsequently fails, causing further deformation of the ankle mortise. The abnormal joint forces resulting from this deformity may ultimately lead to arthritic changes of the hindfoot and midfoot.[30,54]

Recognition of peritalar instability is necessary to provide appropriate management and to stop/prevent further deformation. The clinic visit should start with a thorough clinical examination followed by numerous imaging modalities that can be used to evaluate the medial instability, including conventional plain radiographs, ultrasonography, computed tomography (CT) (including weightbearing CT [WBCT]), and magnetic resonance imaging (MRI). This review article aims to provide a comprehensive understanding of how to interpret and diagnose peritalar instability using each included imaging modality.

CONVENTIONAL PLAIN RADIOGRAPHS

The standard radiographic assessment of the peritalar instability starts with conventional weightbearing radiographs including lateral and mortise views of the ankle, dorsoplantar foot view, and hindfoot alignment view (also known as Saltzman view).[55] Differences in visualized deformity have been reported between weightbearing and non–weightbearing conditions (**Fig. 1**). Therefore, all radiographs should be performed with physiologic loading of the foot to be able to assess the pattern and severity of the underlying deformity most accurately.

Radiographically, peritalar instability can be classified as either varus or valgus, depending on the major direction of the talus tilting in the coronal plane.[56] In either

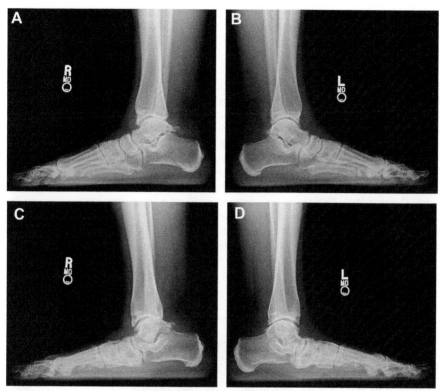

Fig. 1. A 63-year old female patient with chronic bilateral midfoot pain with conventional lateral views of the right (*A*) and left (*A*) foot. Due to persisting pain she was not applying full weightbearing while taking radiographs. True weightbearing lateral views of the right foot (*C*) and left foot (*D*) demonstrate complete collapse of the medial arch in both feet.

scenario, the talus can also present with additional deformity in the sagittal or the axial plane, including the internal or external rotation of the talus relative to the calcaneus. For better understanding of these complex and often 3-dimensional deformities, Hintermann and colleagues[1,2,57] proposed a classification system of peritalar instability that consists of the 2 main deformity types: valgus versus varus deformity. Each group includes subgroups that define the sagittal and axial orientation of the talus resulting in a total of 9 valgus and 9 varus deformity subtypes (**Fig. 2**).[56] Using this system, every

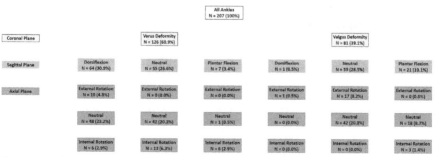

Fig. 2. Classification system of peritalar instability considering all 3 planes.[56]

	All Ankles N = 207 (100%)					
Coronal Plane	**Varus Deformity** N = 126 (60.9%)			**Valgus Deformity** N = 81 (39.1%)		
Sagittal Plane	Dorsiflexion N = 64 (30.9%)	Neutral N = 55 (26.6%)	Plantar Flexion N = 7 (3.4%)	Dorsiflexion N = 1 (0.5%)	Neutral N = 59 (28.5%)	Plantar Flexion N = 21 (10.1%)
Axial Plane	External Rotation N = 10 (4.8%)	External Rotation N = 0 (0.0%)	External Rotation N = 0 (0.0%)	External Rotation N = 1 (0.5%)	External Rotation N = 17 (8.2%)	External Rotation N = 0 (0.0%)
	Neutral N = 48 (23.2%)	Neutral N = 42 (20.3%)	Neutral N = 1 (0.5%)	Neutral N = 0 (0.0%)	Neutral N = 42 (20.3%)	Neutral N = 18 (8.7%)
	Internal Rotation N = 6 (2.9%)	Internal Rotation N = 13 (6.3%)	Internal Rotation N = 6 (2.9%)	Internal Rotation N = 0 (0.0%)	Internal Rotation N = 0 (0.0%)	Internal Rotation N = 3 (1.4%)

deformity can be classified in all 3 planes relative to adjacent bony structures, as delineated by the following parameters.

Coronal Plane

The tibiotalar surface (TTS) angle is the most commonly used parameter to evaluate talar malalignment in the coronal plane (**Fig. 3**A).[56,58–60] This angle is measured between the longitudinal tibial axis and the articular surface of the talar dome of a weightbearing ankle using either an anteroposterior (AP)[61] or mortise view[56] (measured on the medial side). The longitudinal tibial axis is formed by a line bisecting the tibia at 8 and 13 cm above the tibial plafond. The quantitative definition of a normal TTS angle has slightly varied in the prior literature. Hayashi and colleagues[61] reported a mean value of 87.2 ± 2.8° in their normal control group (consisting of 62 ankles in 50 subjects). Comparably, Nosewicz and colleagues[56] described the mean value to be 89.0 ± 2.6° in their study (30 feet) and defined a pathologic valgus tilt as a TTS angle of more than 94.2°. An abnormal valgus tilt on weightbearing AP or mortise radiographs may indicate substantial failure of the deltoid ligament.[62]

The inframalleolar alignment is usually assessed by measurement of calcaneal moment arm using weightbearing hindfoot alignment view (also known as Saltzman

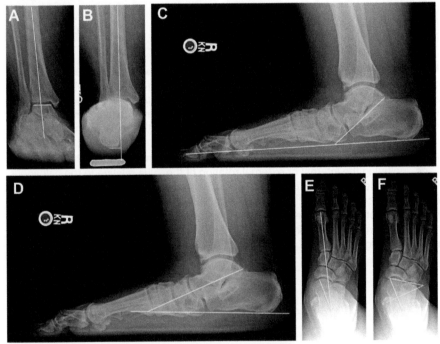

Fig. 3. Conventional weightbearing radiographs of a 50-year-old woman with pes planovalgus et abductus deformity with PTTD grade II. (*A*) Tibiotalar surface measured on mortise view of the ankle (in this case 96°). (*B*) Calcaneal moment arm measured on hindfoot alignment view (in this case 29 mm of valgus). (*C*) Talocalcaneal inclination angle on lateral view of the foot (in this case 39°). (*D*) Talocalcaneal angle on lateral view of the foot (in this case 25°). (*E*) Talometatarsal I angle on dorsoplantar view of the foot (in this case 15°). (*F*) Talonavicular coverage angle on dorsoplantar view of the foot (in this case 36°).

view) (**Fig. 3**B).[55] In patients with subtalar compensation the calcaneal moment can be neutral despite valgus tilting of the talus.[60]

Sagittal Plane

Two parameters have been used to detect the sagittal plane malalignment of the talus including talocalcaneal inclination (TCI) angle and talocalcaneal angle. The TCI angle is measured using the lateral ankle view on weightbearing radiographs (**Fig. 3**C). The TCI angle is defined as the angle formed between a line connecting the talar axis (posterior to anterior talar articular surface at the underside of the talar head) and a line representing the base of the foot (from the inferior aspect of the calcaneal tuberosity to the base of the first metatarsal head).[56,58,63] Nosewicz and colleagues[58] described the normal value of this angle to be $30.5 \pm 4.5°$ in their control group (30 feet), whereas in patients with valgus deformity this value was significantly higher with $36.3 \pm 7.2°$. The talocalcaneal angle is formed by the bisection of the line showing the axis of the talus and a line tangential to the inferior aspect of the calcaneus demonstrating the calcaneal inclination axis (**Fig. 3**D).[52,53,58,64–67] The range of the normal talocalcaneal angle is between 25° and 55°, whereas the angle of more than 55° indicates a valgus alignment of the hindfoot or calcaneus.[68] Steiner and colleagues[53] performed a combined subtalar and naviculocuneiform arthrodesis in 31 patients (34 feet) with PCFD with medial arch collapse at the level of the naviculocuneiform joint. At the 2-year follow-up, the lateral talocalcaneal angle improved from a mean of 39.2° (range, 14.8° to 61.1°) to a mean of 32.2° (range, 17.3° to 43.5°) (P<.001).[53]

Axial Plane

Talometatarsal I angle is defined as the angle between the first metatarsal axis and the talar axis measured on the dorsoplantar foot view on weightbearing radiographs (**Fig. 3**E).[69] A statistically significant difference has been observed between PCFD and control patients with 21.4° versus 7.9°, respectively (P<.001).[69] Talonavicular coverage angle is formed by the bisection of the lines connecting the rims of the articular surfaces of the talus and navicular bone (**Fig. 3**F).[53,65,67,70–74] Similar to the talometatarsal I angle, this parameter also has been demonstrated to be significantly different between PCFD and control patients with 29.9° versus 10.6°, respectively (P<.001).[69]

Although these delineated parameters can provide a thorough assessment of the talar instability in all 3 planes, some concerns may remain regarding their relationship to symptoms. It has been shown that the severity of these parameters may not reliably predict symptoms; however, it has been reported that deformity is likely to be more severe among symptomatic patients in comparison with an asymptomatic cohort.[62] In a retrospective case-control study comparing 50 patients with versus without symptoms, the average talonavicular angle measures on weightbearing AP radiographs was 25° and 38° in patients without and with symptoms, respectively.[62] Furthermore, the weightbearing AP may underestimate the extent of abduction if the patients holds up their arch while the radiograph is taken or if positioning does not allow full weightbearing with the lower leg directly over the foot.[62] Thus, it is recommended to evaluate the patient's clinical alignment while standing for more accurate interpretation what is seen radiographically.

Personal Experience

In our personal experience, the conventional weightbearing radiographs are together with through clinical assessment are the 2 most important tools and available tools for correct assessment of the PCFD. It is crucial that the radiographs are done in standing position. Radiographs should not be older than 6 months at the time of clinical assessment. If in the past 6 months a substantial progression of underlying deformity and/or trauma of foot/ankle was reported, then new radiographs should be obtained. Conventional radiographs should be used for preoperative surgery planning as well as follow-up controls to assess the amount of correction achieved by the surgery.

COMPUTED TOMOGRAPHY/WEIGHTBEARING COMPUTED TOMOGRAPHY

Conventional weightbearing radiographs are imaging of the first choice in patients with PCFD. However, due to complexity of the anatomy and deformity, some interpretation of findings may be challenging. The WBCT is rapidly expanding[75–77] and may allow a more detailed and correct understanding of this complex and 3-dimensional deformity.[30,76,78–91] As in conventional radiographs, weightbearing status has been shown to elicit considerably different measurement in CT as well. De Cesar Netto and colleagues[83] demonstrated that 18 of 19 measurements used for assessment of pes planovalgus deformity significantly different between weightbearing and non–weightbearing CT images (**Table 1**). WBCT is recommended to be used for detailed assessment of PCFD as recently stated by Expert Consensus on PCFD.[30] The following parameters have been used to evaluate the underlying deformities including peritalar instability in patients with PCFD using WBCT (**Fig. 4**).

Coronal Plane

Middle facet subluxation: PCFD may present with substantial subluxation of the subtalar joint (**Fig. 5**).[30,76,81,86,92–95] The deformity can be noted by the decreased overlap/congruence of the anterior, middle, and/or posterior facet of the talus and the calcaneus in patients with symptomatic PCFD. Already in 1999, it has been demonstrated using simulated WBCT that patients with PCFD have decreased congruence of the posterior facet of the subtalar joint in comparison to healthy controls with 68% ± 9% versus 92% ± 2%, respectively ($P = .0066$), as well as of the anterior and middle facets with 51% ± 23% versus 95% ± 6%, respectively ($P = .0066$).[92] Following a protocol similar to what has been described previously,[69,81,96] sagittal WBCT cuts can be used to identify the anterior and posterior edges of the middle facet. The coronal plane images are then used to measure the midpoint position in the anterior-to-posterior plane of the middle talar facet. Then, the percentage of talar of the talar articular surface that is not overlapped by the opposing calcaneal surface is measured (the amount of subluxation, reported as the percentage of "un-coverage") as well as the angle between both articular surfaces (incongruence angle). De Cesar Netto and colleagues[82] found that the middle facet demonstrated significantly increased peritalar subluxation in patients with PCFD in comparison to healthy controls with a mean value of joint un-coverage of 45.3% (95% confidence interval [CI] 38.5%–52.1%) versus 4.8% (95% CI 3.2%–6.4%), respectively ($P<.0001$). A significant difference was also found in the incongruence angle between both groups with a mean angle of 17.3° (95% CI 14.7°–19.9°) versus 0.3° (95% CI 0.1°–0.5°), respectively ($P<.0001$). A critical value of joint incongruence angle of greater than 8.4° was reported to be diagnostic for symptomatic PCFD.[82]

Inftal-hor angle[69]: An angle taken between lines modeling the inferior articular surface of the talus within the posterior subtalar joint and floor (horizontal plane). Inftal-suptal angle[69]: An angle taken between lines modeling the inferior and superior articular surfaces of the talus within the posterior subtalar joint. These 2 angles were found to be significantly greater in patients with PCFD in comparison to a healthy cohort at all 3 locations along the posterior facet of the subtalar joint (25%, 50%, and 75%).[69]

Table 1
Computed tomography–based measurement of progressive collapsing foot deformity

Measurement	NWB Assessment	WB Assessment	Difference in Means	P Value
Axial view				
Talus-first metatarsal angle (°) (see **Fig. 4A**)	13 (10–15)	20 (17–23)	7.2 (3.6–11)	<.0001
Talonavicular coverage angle (°) (see **Fig. 4B**)	21 (18–24)	30 (27–34)	9.1 (4.4–14)	.0002
Coronal view				
Calcaneofibular distance (mm) (see **Fig. 4C**)	6 (5.5–6.5)	5 (4.5–5.5)	−4.5 (−5.9–3.1)	<.0001
Medial cuneiform-to-skin distance (mm) (see **Fig. 4D**)	20 (19–21)	16 (15–17)	−6.2 (−8.1 to −4.3)	<.0001
Navicular-to-skin distance (mm) (see **Fig. 4E**)	25 (24–26)	19 (17–20)	−11 (−13 to −9.1)	<.0001
Medial cuneiform-to-floor distance (mm) (see **Fig. 4F**)	29 (28–31)	18 (17–19)	−15 (−18 to −12)	<.0001
Navicular-to-floor distance (mm) (see **Fig. 4G**)	38 (36–40)	23 (22–25)	−10 (−13 to −8)	<.0001
Subtalar horizontal angle, 25% (°) (see **Fig. 4H**)	23 (22–24)	25 (24–27)	−1.0 (−1.7 to −0.3)	.0035
Subtalar horizontal angle, 50% (°) (see **Fig. 4I**)	15 (14–16)	18 (16–20)	3.0 (0.8–5.2)	.0070
Subtalar horizontal angle, 75% (°) (see **Fig. 4J**)	10 (8.3–11)	13 (11–15)	3.5 (0.9–6.1)	.0070
Forefoot arch angle (°) (see **Fig. 4K**)	13 (12–15)	3 (1.4–4.6)	2.2 (0.2–4.2)	.0310
Sagittal view				
Cuboid-to-skin distance (mm) (see **Fig. 4L**)	20 (19–21)	16 (15–17)	−4.1 (−5.4 to −2.8)	<.0001
Cuboid-to-floor distance (mm)	22 (21–23)	17 (16–18)	−5.3 (−6.8 to −3.8)	<.0001
Medial cuneiform-to-skin distance (mm) (see **Fig. 4M**)	20 (19–22)	16 (15–17)	−4.8 (−6.3 to −3.3)	<.0001
Medial cuneiform-to-floor distance (mm) (see **Fig. 4N**)	29 (27–31)	18 (17–19)	−10.9 (−13 to −8.7)	<.0001
Navicular-to-skin distance (mm) (see **Fig. 4O**)	26 (25–28)	19 (18–21)	−7.2 (−9.6 to −4.8)	<.0001
Navicular-to-floor distance (mm) (see **Fig. 4P**)	38 (36–40)	23 (22–25)	−15 (−17 to −12)	<.0001
Calcaneal inclination angle (°)	16 (15–17)	15 (14–16)	9.8 (7.2–12)	<.0001
Talus-first metatarsal angle (°) (see **Fig. 4Q**)	14 (13–16)	24 (22–26)	−1.1 (−2.6–0.4)	.1446

Values are given as mean with 95% confidence interval.[83]
Abbreviations: NWB, non–weightbearing; WB, weightbearing.

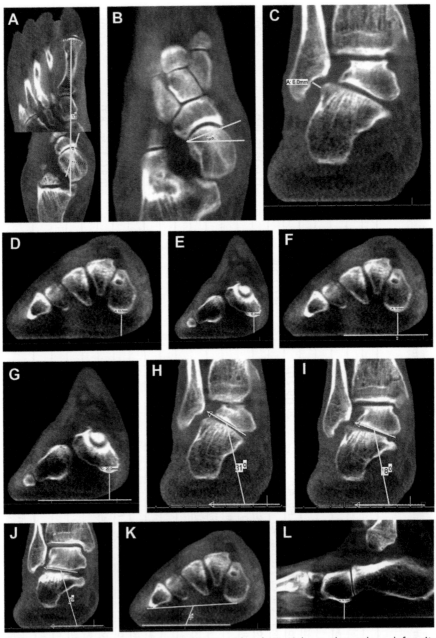

Fig. 4. WBCT in a 54-year old female patient with substantial pes planovalgus deformity. Measurements in axial plane: (*A*) talus-first metatarsal angle (in this case 11°); (*B*) talonavicular coverage angle (in this case 18°). Measurements in coronal plane: (*C*) calcaneofibular distance (in this case 6 mm); (*D*) medial cuneiform-to-skin distance (in this case 14 mm); (*E*) navicular-to-skin distance (in this case 15 mm); (*F*) medial cuneiform-to-floor distance (in this case 14 mm); (*G*) navicular-to-floor distance (in this case 20 mm); (*H*) subtalar horizontal angle, 25% (in this case 31°); (*I*) subtalar horizontal angle, 50% (in this case 18°); (*J*) subtalar horizontal angle, 75% (in this case 8°); (*K*) forefoot arch angle (in this case

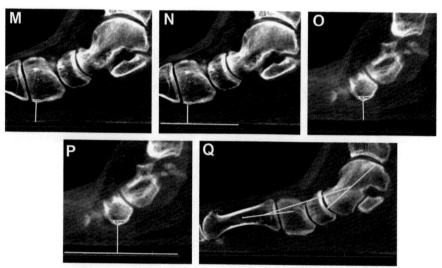

Fig. 4. (*continued*).

Furthermore, a more valgus orientation of the subtalar joint in the PCFD group was observed, which generally increased when measured at different planes from anterior to posterior.[69]

Sagittal Plane

Talus-first metatarsal angle[83]: This angle is formed by the intersection of the longitudinal axis of the first metatarsal and talus. Values are considered positive when the angle had a plantar vertex. De Cesar Netto and colleagues[83] demonstrated this angle has a mean value of 14° (95% CI 13°–16°) versus 24° (95% CI 22°–26°) in patients with PCFD under weightbearing versus non–weightbearing conditions, respectively (see **Table 1**).[83]

Axial Plane

Talus-first metatarsal angle[83]: The axial plane was defined as being parallel to the horizontal platform, with the horizontal edge of the images aligned with the axis of the first metatarsal. This angle is formed by the intersection of the lines representing the axis of the first metatarsal and the axis of the talus. Values are considered positive when the angle had a medial vertex, indicating a relative increase in forefoot abduction. De Cesar Netto and colleagues[83] demonstrated this angle has a mean value of 13° (95% CI 10°–15°) versus 20° (95% CI 17°–23°) in patients with PCFD under weightbearing versus non–weightbearing conditions, respectively (see **Table 1**).[83]

Talonavicular coverage angle[83]: This angle was originally described by Sangeorzan and colleagues[97] that includes angular measurement based on the relationship of the

2°). Measurements in sagittal plane: (*L*) cuboid-to-floor distance (in this case 14 mm); (*M*) medial cuneiform-to-skin distance (in this case 14 mm); (*N*) medial cuneiform-to-floor distance (in this case 15 mm); (*O*) navicular-to-skin distance (in this case 15 mm); (*P*) navicular-to-floor distance (in this case 20 mm); and (*Q*) talus-first metatarsal angle (in this case 33°).

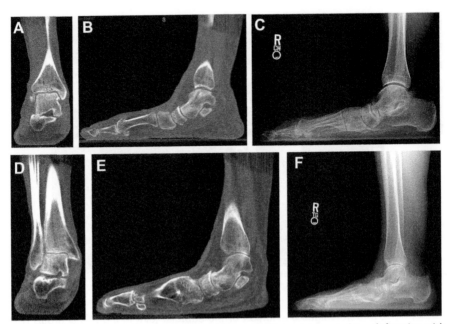

Fig. 5. (A) A 54-year-old female patient with substantial pes planovalgus deformity with concomitant middle facet subluxation as seen on coronal plane of WBCT. Also, substantial degeneration of the subtalar joint is present. (B) Sagittal plane of WBCT and (C) weightbearing lateral view of the foot demonstrate substantial break-down of the medial arch at the level of the naviculocuneiform joint. (D) A 62-year old male patient with substantial pes planovalgus with well-preserved congruity of the middle facet of the subtalar joint. (E) Sagittal plane of WBCT and (F) weightbearing lateral view of the foot demonstrate substantial break-down of the medial arch at the level of the naviculocuneiform joint.

center of the talus to the center of the navicular. In their study using conventional 2-dimensional imaging, they observed a significant improvement of the talonavicular coverage angle by 26% following lateral calcaneal lengthening osteotomy in patients with PCFD.[97] In WBCT, De Cesar Netto and colleagues[83] demonstrated this angle has a mean value of 21° (95% CI 18°–24°) versus 30° (95% CI 27°–34°) in patients with PCFD under weightbearing versus non–weightbearing conditions, respectively (see **Table 1**).[83]

Personal Experience

Although weightbearing conventional radiographs are mandatory for radiographic assessment of the PCFD, WBCT should be performed additionally if available. This has been recently suggested by the expert consensus recently published in *Foot & Ankle International*.[76,98] Conventional radiographs can provide important information to estimate the underlying deformity; however, it is limited to 2-dimensional analysis. WBCT can provide additional information such as true alignment of the subtalar joint including medial and posterior facets, presence of subfibular and/or sinus tarsi impingement, subluxation of the subtalar joint at the posterior and/or middle facet, and extent of degeneration of the subtalar and talonavicular joint with true joint space visible. Especially newer investigations demonstrate that the middle facet subluxation may be an earlier and more sensitive marker of deformity progression rather than changes around the posterior facet of the subtalar joint.[81] In our opinion, only WBCT can provide detailed information of all aspects of underlying PCFD. However, it is obvious that the access to the WBCT imaging is still quite limited. Recently, de Cesar Netto and colleagues[99] analyzed both WBCT and MRI in patients with flexible PCFD. The main results from this study were (1) sinus tarsi impingement on WBCT was associated with degenerative changes of posterior tibial tendon (PTT) on MRI, (2) patients with subtalar joint subluxation often demonstrated pathologic findings of the spring ligament, and (3) subfibular impingement on WBCT statistically correlated with talocalcaneal interosseous involvement on MRI.[99] Of course, MRI can and should not replace WBCT; however, it may give important information as mentioned previously.

MAGNETIC RESONANCE IMAGING

The MRI is widely recognized as the gold standard for assessing soft tissue pathology by direct evaluation of the tissue's configuration and integrity.[100–111] However, the inability to regularly obtain an evaluation under weightbearing conditions distorts the true presentation of the peritalar deformity and prevents investigators from drawing a confident correlation between the degree of injury in each part of the medial ligamentous complex on MRI and its resultant instability. Despite of correlation of some alignment parameters,[112] in patients with PCFD MRI should be used to assess the integrity of periarticular structures including deltoid ligament (**Fig. 6**), spring ligament (**Fig. 7**), and PTT (**Fig. 8**)[113] and not for assessment of underlying midfoot and hindfoot alignment.

The deltoid ligament is composed of both deep and superficial layers.[14,15] Typically, the deep layer includes the anterior tibiotalar ligament and the more robust posterior tibiotalar ligament; these structures work in tandem to stabilize the tibiotalar articulation by resisting ankle valgus. The longer superficial deltoid ligaments normally include the tibionavicular and tibiospring ligaments, which span the talonavicular joint; the tibiocalcaneal ligament, which spans the subtalar joint; and the superficial tibiotalar ligament, which spans the ankle joint. However, anatomic variations in the components of each layer have been previously described.[7,15,114–120] Kelikian and Sarrafian[7] mentioned 13 different anatomic descriptions published between 1822 and 1979. Panchani and colleagues[118] found 8 different bands of the deltoid ligament; 6 of 8, as mentioned previously, were more frequently encountered than the 2 additional variants (a band deep to the tibiocalcaneal ligament and a band posterior to sustentaculum tali). Conversely, Campbell and colleagues[116] only reported the tibionavicular, tibiospring, and deep posterior tibiotalar ligament bands as 3 constant components of the deltoid ligament.

In patients with PCFD, the ability of the tibionavicular and tibiospring ligaments, that normally stabilize the talonavicular joint by limiting hindfoot eversion and inward displacement of the talar head, is limited due to irregularities of the deltoid ligament. In addition, further damage to the deep deltoid ligament can occur late in this process, allowing the tibiotalar joint to tilt into valgus, contributing to a hindfoot valgus deformity. In the assessment of the deltoid ligament using MRI, axial and coronal views are of most use for distinguishing its various components, which appear as low-to intermediate-signal-intensity bands that broaden distally. Signal intensity becomes heterogeneous as the age of the patient increases, and by itself, should not be used as a reliable indicator of ligament irregularity. Aside from this exception, the loss of normal fatty striations, signal intensity heterogeneity, and architectural distortion indicate degeneration, low-grade tearing, and fibrosis. This interpretation should be distinct from that of high-grade tearing, which produces large fluid-filled gaps or frank

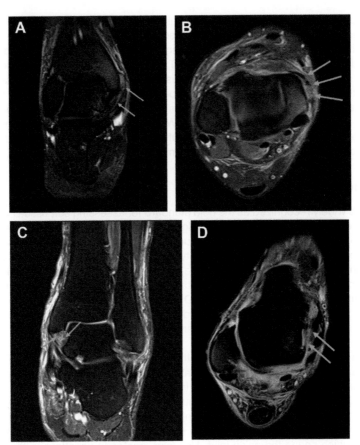

Fig. 6. MRI of the deltoid ligament. (*A*) Coronal T2 fat-saturated (FS) and (*B*) axial proton density (PD) FS images demonstrate tear of the superficial deltoid ligament and stripping from the medial malleolus (*arrows*). (*C*) Coronal T2 FS imaging demonstrates a tear of the deep deltoid ligament (*arrow*) with loss of the normal architecture and increased signal. (*D*) Axial PD FS imaging demonstrates tear of the deep deltoid ligament (*arrow*) with loss of the normal architecture and increased signal.

discontinuity. High-grade deep deltoid ligamentous tears more commonly result from trauma and are related to chronic PCFD.[22]

Quantitatively, Ormsby and colleagues[108] described an important role of the tibionavicular ligament in PCFD. They found that when viewed on the novel oblique axial view, the ligament had a mean length of 15.4 mm, with a homogeneous mean width of 7.3 mm at its origin and 6.6 mm at its insertion. It was homogeneous black or gray/black, with longitudinal stripes of mildly increased signal. Sagittally, on both T1-weighted and T2-weighted images, the ligament was viewed as a homogeneous black structure, with a mean length of 14.7 mm and thickness of 2.3 mm. In the group with known irregularities of the talonavicular ligament, the structure was thickened proximally, with distal attenuation and intrasubstance edema. Five patients (5 of 9, 55.6%) from this group underwent corrective surgery, where no patients in the normal group had correction performed.[108]

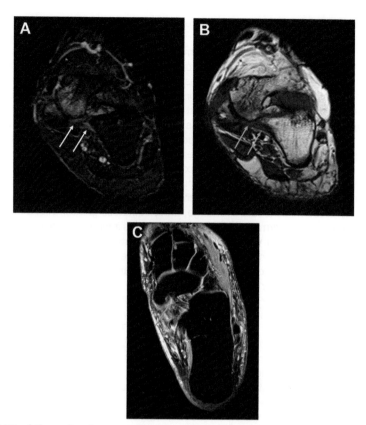

Fig. 7. MRI of the spring ligament. (*A*) Coronal T2 FS and (*B*) coronal T1 imaging demonstrates partial tear of the spring ligament (*arrows*) with increased signal (T2 FS) and loss of normal periligamentous fat (T1). (*C*) Axial PD FS showing tear of the calcaneospring (superomedial calcaneonavicular) ligament from the navicular attachment.

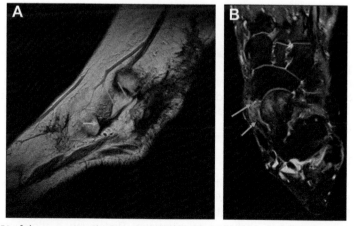

Fig. 8. MRI of the posterior tibial tendon (PTT). (*A*) Sagittal PD imaging demonstrates a near complete tear of the PTT (*blue arrow*) just proximal to the navicular attachment (*green arrow*). (*B*) Axial PD FS imaging demonstrates a tear of the PTT (*blue arrow*) from the navicular attachment and mild tendon stump (*green arrow*) retraction.

The spring ligament complex is another important structure that may contribute substantially to progression of PCFD.[17,31,34,72,121–128] It usually consists of 3 portions, from medial to lateral: the superomedial, medioplantar oblique, and inferoplantar longitudinal bundles.[35,106,129,130] The superomedial bundle, the largest bundle of the complex, arises from the superomedial sustentaculum tali and passes below the talus and navicular tuberosity before its insertion on the distal superomedial navicular. This bundle forms a hammocklike structure that supports the talar head, talonavicular joint, and separates the PTT from the talus. It is challenging to assess the spring ligament clinically; thus, imaging is valuable to adequately evaluate this structure. All components of the spring ligament are well delineated on a high-field MRI. The superomedial bundle is best visualized on coronal and axial oblique planes. It appears as a 2-mm to 5-mm smooth, low-signal-intensity structure that is continuous with the superficial deltoid ligament. A spring ligament abnormality is most commonly seen in this bundle and typically presents as a caliber change; band thickness greater than 5 mm or less than 2 mm indicates abnormality.[106] Additional findings include increased signal intensity, ligament elongation or waviness, fiber discontinuity, and periligamentous edema that is typically focused at the distal ligament. A complete tear allows the PTT to come in contact with the talar head directly, without any separating tissue. The medioplantar oblique and inferoplantar longitudinal bundles are best seen in the axial plane. Any abnormality of these 2 smaller plantar bundles is less common, more challenging to diagnose, and rarely addressed surgically. The spring ligament lesion is often associated with substantial degeneration/injury of PTT as it has been demonstrated in the study by Balen and Helms[131] with up to 92%. Deland and colleagues[132] analyzed MRI in 31 consecutive patients with PTTD to assess the involvement of medial ligament in pathologic process. Two groups were assessed, patients with PCFD versus healthy controls. Statistically significant differences between both groups were found for the superomedial calcaneonavicular ligament ($P<.0001$), inferomedial calcaneonavicular ligament ($P<.0001$), interosseus ligament ($P = .0009$), anterior component of the superficial deltoid ($P<.0001$), plantar metatarsal ligament ($P = .0002$), and plantar naviculocuneiform ligament ($P = .0006$). Three ligaments with the most severe degenerative changes were the spring ligament complex (superomedial and inferomedial calcaneonavicular ligaments) and the talocalcaneal interosseous ligament.[132]

Personal Experience

It is still uncertain whether medial soft tissue reconstruction including deltoid and spring ligaments as well as PTT should be additionally performed with osseous correction of the underlying deformity.[121,133] Therefore, MRI can be of value in patients with clinical suspicion of damage/degeneration of deltoid and spring ligament and/or PTT for appropriate preoperative planning to add these surgical steps into the PCFD correction.

SUMMARY

Undiagnosed medial ankle instability can be a prerequisite for pathogenic progression in the foot, particularly for PCFD. With the complex anatomy in this region, and the limitations of each individual investigational method, accurately identifying peritalar instability remains a serious challenge to clinicians. Performing a thorough clinical examination aided by evaluation with advanced imaging can improve the threshold of detection for this condition and allow early proper treatment to prevent further manifestations of the instability.

CLINICS CARE POINTS

- Keep in mind that peritalar instability has several facets of appearance so the appropriate diagnosis is quite challenging.
- Start always with a through clinical examination.
- Use different imaging modalities if needed.
- As of now, only weightbearing computed tomography reliably reveals all aspects of complex peritalad deformity.
- Use magnetic resonance imaging for detailed assessment of soft tissue structures on the medial side of the foot and hindfoot.

DISCLOSURE

The authors declared no potential conflicts of interest with respect to the research, authorship, and/or publication of this article.

ACKNOWLEDGMENTS

The authors thank Dr Megan K. Mills, MD (Department of Radiology and Imaging Sciences, University of Utah) and Jesse Steadman, BS (Department of Orthopedics, University of Utah) for their outstanding help and support to identify the patients with peritalar instability in our department and to prepare the clinical figures.

REFERENCES

1. Hintermann B, Knupp M, Barg A. Peritalar instability. Foot Ankle Int 2012;33(5): 450–4.
2. Hintermann B, Knupp M, Barg A. Joint-preserving surgery of asymmetric ankle osteoarthritis with peritalar instability. Foot Ankle Clin 2013;18(3):503–16.
3. Barg A, Pagenstert GI, Hugle T, et al. Ankle osteoarthritis: Etiology, diagnostics, and classification. Foot Ankle Clin 2013;18(3):411–26.
4. Lee WC, Moon JS, Lee HS, et al. Alignment of ankle and hindfoot in early stage ankle osteoarthritis. Foot Ankle Int 2011;32(7):693–9.
5. Bartoníček J, Rammelt S, Naňka O. Anatomy of the subtalar joint. Foot Ankle Clin 2018;23(3):315–40.
6. Cody EA, Williamson ER, Burket JC, et al. Correlation of talar anatomy and subtalar joint alignment on weightbearing computed tomography with radiographic flatfoot parameters. Foot Ankle Int 2016;37(8):874–81.
7. Kelikian AS, Sarrafian SK. Sarrafian's anatomy of the foot and ankle: Descriptive, topographic, functional. Philadelphia: Lippincott Williams & Wilkins; 2011.
8. Krahenbuhl N, Horn-Lang T, Hintermann B, et al. The subtalar joint: A complex mechanism. EFORT Open Rev 2017;2(7):309–16.
9. Maceira E, Monteagudo M. Subtalar anatomy and mechanics. Foot Ankle Clin 2015;20(2):195–221.
10. Sangeorzan A, Sangeorzan B. Subtalar joint biomechanics: From normal to pathologic. Foot Ankle Clin 2018;23(3):341–52.
11. Hintermann B, Nigg BM, Sommer C. Foot movement and tendon excursion: An in vitro study. Foot Ankle Int 1994;15(7):386–95.
12. Rammelt S, Zwipp H. Talar neck and body fractures. Injury 2009;40(2):120–35.

13. Burks RT, Morgan J. Anatomy of the lateral ankle ligaments. Am J Sports Med 1994;22(1):72–7.

14. Golano P, Vega J, De Leeuw PA, et al. Anatomy of the ankle ligaments: A pictorial essay. Knee Surg Sports Traumatol Arthrosc 2016;24(4):944–56.

15. Hintermann B, Golano P. The anatomy and function of the deltoid ligament. Tech Foot Ankle 2014;13(2):67–72.

16. Oburu E, Myerson MS. Deltoid ligament repair in flatfoot deformity. Foot Ankle Clin 2017;22(3):503–14.

17. Salat P, Le V, Veljkovic A, et al. Imaging in foot and ankle instability. Foot Ankle Clin 2018;23(4):499–522.e8.

18. Acevedo JI, Mangone P. Ankle instability and arthroscopic lateral ligament repair. Foot Ankle Clin 2015;20(1):59–69.

19. Acevedo JI, Palmer RC, Mangone PG. Arthroscopic treatment of ankle instability: Brostrom. Foot Ankle Clin 2018;23(4):555–70.

20. Alshalawi S, Galhoum AE, Alrashidi Y, et al. Medial ankle instability: The deltoid dilemma. Foot Ankle Clin 2018;23(4):639–57.

21. Glazebrook M, Eid M, Alhadhoud M, et al. Percutaneous ankle reconstruction of lateral ligaments. Foot Ankle Clin 2018;23(4):581–92.

22. Hintermann B. Medial ankle instability. Foot Ankle Clin 2003;8(4):723–38.

23. Hintermann B, Knupp M, Pagenstert GI. Deltoid ligament injuries: Diagnosis and management. Foot Ankle Clin 2006;11(3):625–37.

24. Hintermann B, Valderrabano V, Boss A, et al. Medial ankle instability: An exploratory, prospective study of fifty-two cases. Am J Sports Med 2004;32(1):183–90.

25. Mittlmeier T, Rammelt S. Update on subtalar joint instability. Foot Ankle Clin 2018;23(3):397–413.

26. O'neil JT, Guyton GP. Revision of surgical lateral ankle ligament stabilization. Foot Ankle Clin 2018;23(4):605–24.

27. Porter DA, Kamman KA. Chronic lateral ankle instability: Open surgical management. Foot Ankle Clin 2018;23(4):539–54.

28. Slater K. Acute lateral ankle instability. Foot Ankle Clin 2018;23(4):523–37.

29. Teixeira J, Guillo S. Arthroscopic treatment of ankle instability - Allograft/autograft reconstruction. Foot Ankle Clin 2018;23(4):571–9.

30. Myerson MS, Thordarson DB, Johnson JE, et al. Classification and nomenclature: progressive collapsing foot deformity. Foot Ankle Int 2020;41(10):1271–6.

31. Bastias GF, Dalmau-Pastor M, Astudillo C, et al. Spring ligament instability. Foot Ankle Clin 2018;23(4):659–78.

32. Deland JT. The adult acquired flatfoot and spring ligament complex. Pathology and implications for treatment. Foot Ankle Clin 2001;6(1):129–35.

33. Golano P, Farinas O, Saenz I. The anatomy of the navicular and periarticular structures. Foot Ankle Clin 2004;9(1):1–23.

34. Steginsky B, Vora A. What to do with the spring ligament. Foot Ankle Clin 2017; 22(3):515–27.

35. Taniguchi A, Tanaka Y, Takakura Y, et al. Anatomy of the spring ligament. J Bone Joint Surg Am 2003;85-a(11):2174–8.

36. Haleem AM, Pavlov H, Bogner E, et al. Comparison of deformity with respect to the talus in patients with posterior tibial tendon dysfunction and controls using multiplanar weight-bearing imaging or conventional radiography. J Bone Joint Surg Am 2014;96(8):e63.

37. Mosier-Laclair S, Pomeroy G, Manoli A 2nd. Operative treatment of the difficult stage 2 adult acquired flatfoot deformity. Foot Ankle Clin 2001;6(1):95–119.

38. Myerson MS. Adult acquired flatfoot deformity: Treatment of dysfunction of the posterior tibial tendon. Instr Course Lect 1997;46:393–405.

39. Röhm J, Zwicky L, Horn Lang T, et al. Mid- to long-term outcome of 96 corrective hindfoot fusions in 84 patients with rigid flatfoot deformity. Bone Joint J 2015; 97-b(5):668–74.

40. Sizensky JA, Marks RM. Medial-sided bony procedures: Why, what, and how? Foot Ankle Clin 2003;8(3):539–62.

41. Zhang YJ, Du JY, Chen B, et al. Correlation between three-dimensional medial longitudinal arch joint complex mobility and medial arch angle in stage II posterior tibial tendon dysfunction. Foot Ankle Surg 2019;25(6):721–6.

42. Zhang YJ, Xu J, Wang Y, et al. Correlation between hindfoot joint three-dimensional kinematics and the changes of the medial arch angle in stage II posterior tibial tendon dysfunction flatfoot. Clin Biomech (Bristol, Avon) 2015; 30(2):153–8.

43. Heilman AE, Braly WG, Bishop JO, et al. An anatomic study of subtalar instability. Foot Ankle 1990;10(4):224–8.

44. Kato T. The diagnosis and treatment of instability of the subtalar joint. J Bone Joint Surg Br 1995;77(3):400–6.

45. Ringleb SI, Dhakal A, Anderson CD, et al. Effects of lateral ligament sectioning on the stability of the ankle and subtalar joint. J Orthop Res 2011;29(10): 1459–64.

46. Tochigi Y. Effect of arch supports on ankle-subtalar complex instability: A biomechanical experimental study. Foot Ankle Int 2003;24(8):634–9.

47. Tochigi Y, Amendola A, Rudert MJ, et al. The role of the interosseous talocalcaneal ligament in subtalar joint stability. Foot Ankle Int 2004;25(8):588–96.

48. Tochigi Y, Takahashi K, Yamagata M, et al. Influence of the interosseous talocalcaneal ligament injury on stability of the ankle-subtalar joint complex–A cadaveric experimental study. Foot Ankle Int 2000;21(6):486–91.

49. Tochigi Y, Yoshinaga K, Wada Y, et al. Acute inversion injury of the ankle: magnetic resonance imaging and clinical outcomes. Foot Ankle Int 1998;19(11): 730–4.

50. Jack EA. Naviculo-cuneiform fusion in the treatment of flat foot. J Bone Joint Surg Br 1953;35-b(1):75–82.

51. Barg A, Brunner S, Zwicky L, et al. Subtalar and naviculocuneiform fusion for extended breakdown of the medial arch. Foot Ankle Clin 2011;16(1):69–81.

52. Hintermann B, Deland JT, De Cesar Netto C, et al. Consensus on indications for isolated subtalar joint fusion and naviculocuneiform fusions for progressive collapsing foot deformity. Foot Ankle Int 2020;41(10):1295–8.

53. Steiner CS, Gilgen A, Zwicky L, et al. Combined subtalar and naviculocuneiform fusion for treating adult acquired flatfoot deformity with medial arch collapse at the level of the naviculocuneiform joint. Foot Ankle Int 2019;40(1):42–7.

54. Bohay DR, Anderson JG. Stage IV posterior tibial tendon insufficiency: The tilted ankle. Foot Ankle Clin 2003;8(3):619–36.

55. Saltzman CL, El-Khoury GY. The hindfoot alignment view. Foot Ankle Int 1995; 16(9):572–6.

56. Nosewicz TL, Knupp M, Bolliger L, et al. Radiological morphology of peritalar instability in varus and valgus tilted ankles. Foot Ankle Int 2014;35(5):453–62.

57. Hintermann B, Knupp M, Barg A. [Joint preserving surgery in patients with peritalar instability]. Fuss Sprungg 2013;11(4):196–206.

58. Nosewicz TL, Knupp M, Bolliger L, et al. The reliability and validity of radiographic measurements for determining the three-dimensional position of the

talus in varus and valgus osteoarthritic ankles. Skeletal Radiol 2012;41(12): 1567–73.

59. Son HS, Choi JG, Ahn J, et al. Hindfoot alignment change after total ankle arthroplasty for varus osteoarthritis. Foot Ankle Int 2020. 1071100720970937.

60. Wang B, Saltzman CL, Chalayon O, et al. Does the subtalar joint compensate for ankle malalignment in end-stage ankle arthritis? Clin Orthop Relat Res 2015; 473(1):318–25.

61. Hayashi K, Tanaka Y, Kumai T, et al. Correlation of compensatory alignment of the subtalar joint to the progression of primary osteoarthritis of the ankle. Foot Ankle Int 2008;29(4):400–6.

62. Deland JT. Adult-acquired flatfoot deformity. J Am Acad Orthop Surg 2008; 16(7):399–406.

63. Colin F, Bolliger L, Horn Lang T, et al. Effect of supramalleolar osteotomy and total ankle replacement on talar position in the varus osteoarthritic ankle: A comparative study. Foot Ankle Int 2014;35(5):445–52.

64. Aebi J, Horisberger M, Frigg A. Radiographic study of pes planovarus. Foot Ankle Int 2017;38(5):526–31.

65. Kara M, Bayram S. Effect of unilateral accessory navicular bone on radiologic parameters of foot. Foot Ankle Int 2020. 1071100720964820.

66. Tsai J, Mcdonald E, Sutton R, et al. Severe flexible pes planovalgus deformity correction using trabecular metallic wedges. Foot Ankle Int 2019;40(4):402–7.

67. Yuan C, Wang C, Zhang C, et al. Derotation of the talus and arthrodesis treatment of stages II-V Müller-Weiss disease: Midterm results of 36 cases. Foot Ankle Int 2019;40(5):506–14.

68. Frances JM, Feldman DS. Management of idiopathic and nonidiopathic flatfoot. Instr Course Lect 2015;64:429–40.

69. Probasco W, Haleem AM, Yu J, et al. Assessment of coronal plane subtalar joint alignment in peritalar subluxation via weight-bearing multiplanar imaging. Foot Ankle Int 2015;36(3):302–9.

70. Bernasconi A, Argyropoulos M, Patel S, et al. Subtalar arthroereisis as an adjunct procedure improves forefoot abduction in stage IIb adult-acquired flatfoot deformity. Foot Ankle Spec 2020. 1938640020951031.

71. Bock P, Pittermann M, Chraim M, et al. The inter- and intraobserver reliability for the radiological parameters of flatfoot, before and after surgery. Bone Joint J 2018;100-b(5):596–602.

72. Brodell JD Jr, Macdonald A, Perkins JA, et al. Deltoid-spring ligament reconstruction in adult acquired flatfoot deformity with medial peritalar instability. Foot Ankle Int 2019;40(7):753–61.

73. Kim J, Day J, Seilern Und Aspang J. Outcomes following revision surgery after failed kidner procedure for painful accessory navicular. Foot Ankle Int 2020; 41(12):1493–501.

74. Willauer P, Sangeorzan BJ, Whittaker EC, et al. The sensitivity of standard radiographic foot measures to misalignment. Foot Ankle Int 2014;35(12):1334–40.

75. Conti MS, Ellis SJ. Weight-bearing CT scans in foot and ankle surgery. J Am Acad Orthop Surg 2020;28(14):e595–603.

76. De Cesar Netto C, Myerson MS, Day J, et al. Consensus for the use of weight-bearing CT in the assessment of progressive collapsing foot deformity. Foot Ankle Int 2020;41(10):1277–82.

77. Lintz F, De Cesar Netto C, Barg A, et al. Weight-bearing cone beam CT scans in the foot and ankle. EFORT Open Rev 2018;3(5):278–86.

78. Burssens A, Barg A, Van Ovost E, et al. The hind- and midfoot alignment computed after a medializing calcaneal osteotomy using a 3D weightbearing CT. Int J Comput Assist Radiol Surg 2019;14(8):1439–47.
79. Day J, De Cesar Netto C, Nishikawa DRC, et al. Three-dimensional biometric weightbearing CT evaluation of the operative treatment of adult-acquired flatfoot deformity. Foot Ankle Int 2020;41(8):930–6.
80. De Cesar Netto C, Bang K, Mansur NS, et al. Multiplanar semiautomatic assessment of foot and ankle offset in adult acquired flatfoot deformity. Foot Ankle Int 2020;41(7):839–48.
81. De Cesar Netto C, Godoy-Santos AL, Saito GH, et al. Subluxation of the middle facet of the subtalar joint as a marker of peritalar subluxation in adult acquired flatfoot deformity: A case-control study. J Bone Joint Surg Am 2019;101(20): 1838–44.
82. De Cesar Netto C, Kunas GC, Soukup D, et al. Correlation of clinical evaluation and radiographic hindfoot alignment in stage II adult-acquired flatfoot deformity. Foot Ankle Int 2018;39(7):771–9.
83. De Cesar Netto C, Schon LC, Thawait GK, et al. Flexible adult acquired flatfoot deformity: comparison between weight-bearing and non-weight-bearing measurements using cone-beam computed tomography. J Bone Joint Surg Am 2017;99(18):e98.
84. De Cesar Netto C, Shakoor D, Dein EJ, et al. Influence of investigator experience on reliability of adult acquired flatfoot deformity measurements using weightbearing computed tomography. Foot Ankle Surg 2019;25(4):495–502.
85. De Cesar Netto C, Shakoor D, Roberts L, et al. Hindfoot alignment of adult acquired flatfoot deformity: A comparison of clinical assessment and weightbearing cone beam CT examinations. Foot Ankle Surg 2018;25(6):790–7.
86. De Cesar Netto C, Silva T, Li S, et al. Assessment of posterior and middle facet subluxation of the subtalar joint in progressive flatfoot deformity. Foot Ankle Int 2020;41(10):1190–7.
87. Jeng CL, Rutherford T, Hull MG, et al. Assessment of bony subfibular impingement in flatfoot patients using weight-bearing CT scans. Foot Ankle Int 2019; 40(2):152–8.
88. Peiffer M, Belvedere C, Clockaerts S, et al. Three-dimensional displacement after a medializing calcaneal osteotomy in relation to the osteotomy angle and hindfoot alignment. Foot Ankle Surg 2020;26(1):78–84.
89. Pilania K, Jankharia B, Monoot P. Role of the weight-bearing cone-beam CT in evaluation of flatfoot deformity. Indian J Radiol Imaging 2019;29(4):364–71.
90. Shakoor D, De Cesar Netto C, Thawait GK, et al. Weight-bearing radiographs and cone-beam computed tomography examinations in adult acquired flatfoot deformity. Foot Ankle Surg 2021;27(2):201–6.
91. Zhang Y, Xu J, Wang X, et al. An in vivo study of hindfoot 3D kinetics in stage II posterior tibial tendon dysfunction (PTTD) flatfoot based on weight-bearing CT scan. Bone Joint Res 2013;2(12):255–63.
92. Ananthakrisnan D, Ching R, Tencer A, et al. Subluxation of the talocalcaneal joint in adults who have symptomatic flatfoot. J Bone Joint Surg Am 1999;81(8): 1147–54.
93. Dullaert K, Hagen JE, Simons P, et al. Influence of tibialis posterior muscle activation on foot anatomy under axial loading: A biomechanical CT human cadaveric study. Foot Ankle Surg 2017;23(4):250–4.
94. Ferri M, Scharfenberger AV, Goplen G, et al. Weightbearing CT scan of severe flexible pes planus deformities. Foot Ankle Int 2008;29(2):199–204.

95. Kunas GC, Probasco W, Haleem AM, et al. Evaluation of peritalar subluxation in adult acquired flatfoot deformity using computed tomography and weightbearing multiplanar imaging. Foot Ankle Surg 2018;24(6):495–500.

96. Apostle KL, Coleman NW, Sangeorzan BJ. Subtalar joint axis in patients with symptomatic peritalar subluxation compared to normal controls. Foot Ankle Int 2014;35(11):1153–8.

97. Sangeorzan BJ, Mosca V, Hansen ST Jr. Effect of calcaneal lengthening on relationships among the hindfoot, midfoot, and forefoot. Foot Ankle 1993;14(3): 136–41.

98. De Cesar Netto C, Deland JT, Ellis SJ. Guest editorial: Expert consensus on adult-acquired flatfoot deformity. Foot Ankle Int 2020;41(10):1269–71.

99. De Cesar Netto C, Saito GH, Roney A, et al. Combined weightbearing CT and MRI assessment of flexible progressive collapsing foot deformity. Foot Ankle Surg 2020.

100. Albano D, Martinelli N, Bianchi A, et al. Posterior tibial tendon dysfunction: Clinical and magnetic resonance imaging findings having histology as reference standard. Eur J Radiol 2018;99:55–61.

101. Arnoldner MA, Gruber M, Syré S, et al. Imaging of posterior tibial tendon dysfunction–Comparison of high-resolution ultrasound and 3T MRI. Eur J Radiol 2015;84(9):1777–81.

102. Braito M, Wöß M, Henninger B, et al. Comparison of preoperative MRI and intra-operative findings of posterior tibial tendon insufficiency. Springerplus 2016; 5(1):1414.

103. Deorio JK, Shapiro SA, Mcneil RB, et al. Validity of the posterior tibial edema sign in posterior tibial tendon dysfunction. Foot Ankle Int 2011;32(2):189–92.

104. Dimmick S, Chhabra A, Grujic L, et al. Acquired flat foot deformity: postoperative imaging. Semin Musculoskelet Radiol 2012;16(3):217–32.

105. Lin YC, Mhuircheartaigh JN, Lamb J, et al. Imaging of adult flatfoot: correlation of radiographic measurements with MRI. AJR Am J Roentgenol 2015;204(2): 354–9.

106. Mengiardi B, Pinto C, Zanetti M. Spring ligament complex and posterior tibial tendon: MR anatomy and findings in acquired adult flatfoot deformity. Semin Musculoskelet Radiol 2016;20(1):104–15.

107. Omar H, Saini V, Wadhwa V, et al. Spring ligament complex: Illustrated normal anatomy and spectrum of pathologies on 3T MR imaging. Eur J Radiol 2016; 85(11):2133–43.

108. Ormsby N, Jackson G, Evans P, et al. Imaging of the tibionavicular ligament, and its potential role in adult acquired flatfoot deformity. Foot Ankle Int 2018; 39(5):629–35.

109. Orr JD, Nunley JA 2nd. Isolated spring ligament failure as a cause of adult-acquired flatfoot deformity. Foot Ankle Int 2013;34(6):818–23.

110. Williams G, Widnall J, Evans P, et al. MRI features most often associated with surgically proven tears of the spring ligament complex. Skeletal Radiol 2013; 42(7):969–73.

111. Wong MW, Griffith JF. Magnetic resonance imaging in adolescent painful flexible flatfoot. Foot Ankle Int 2009;30(4):303–8.

112. Haldar A, Bernasconi A, Junaid SE, et al. 3D imaging for hindfoot alignment assessment: A comparative study between non-weight-bearing MRI and weight-bearing CT. Skeletal Radiol 2021;50(1):179–88.

113. Crim J. Medial-sided ankle pain: Deltoid ligament and beyond. Magn Reson Imaging Clin N Am 2017;25(1):63–77.

114. Amaha K, Nimura A, Yamaguchi R, et al. Anatomic study of the medial side of the ankle base on the joint capsule: An alternative description of the deltoid and spring ligament. J Exp Orthop 2019;6(1):2.
115. Boss AP, Hintermann B. Anatomical study of the medial ankle ligament complex. Foot Ankle Int 2002;23(6):547–53.
116. Campbell KJ, Michalski MP, Wilson KJ, et al. The ligament anatomy of the deltoid complex of the ankle: A qualitative and quantitative anatomical study. J Bone Joint Surg Am 2014;96(8):e62.
117. Guerra-Pinto F, Fabian A, Mota T, et al. The tibiocalcaneal bundle of the deltoid ligament - Prevalence and variations. Foot Ankle Surg 2021;27(2):138–42.
118. Panchani PN, Chappell TM, Moore GD, et al. Anatomic study of the deltoid ligament of the ankle. Foot Ankle Int 2014;35(9):916–21.
119. Won HJ, Koh IJ, Won HS. Morphologic variations of the deltoid ligament of the medial ankle. Clin Anat 2016;29(8):1059–65.
120. Yammine K. The morphology and prevalence of the deltoid complex ligament of the ankle. Foot Ankle Spec 2017;10(1):55–62.
121. Deland JT, Ellis SJ, Day J, et al. Indications for deltoid and spring ligament reconstruction in progressive collapsing foot deformity. Foot Ankle Int 2020; 41(10):1302–6.
122. Heyes G, Swanton E, Vosoughi AR, et al. Comparative study of spring ligament reconstructions using either hamstring allograft or synthetic ligament augmentation. Foot Ankle Int 2020;41(7):803–10.
123. Lui TH. Arthroscopic repair of superomedial spring ligament by talonavicular arthroscopy. Arthrosc Tech 2017;6(1):e31–5.
124. Lui TH, Mak CYD. Arthroscopic approach to the spring (calcaneonavicular) ligament. Foot Ankle Surg 2018;24(3):242–5.
125. Macdonald A, Ciufo D, Vess E, et al. Peritalar kinematics with combined deltoid-spring ligament reconstruction in simulated advanced adult acquired flatfoot deformity. Foot Ankle Int 2020;41(9):1149–57.
126. Nery C, Lemos A, Raduan F, et al. Combined spring and deltoid ligament repair in adult-acquired flatfoot. Foot Ankle Int 2018;39(8):903–7.
127. Ryssman DB, Jeng CL. Reconstruction of the spring ligament with a posterior tibial tendon autograft: Technique tip. Foot Ankle Int 2017;38(4):452–6.
128. Tang CYK, Ng KH. A valuable option: clinical and radiological outcomes of braided suture tape system augmentation for spring ligament repair in flexible flatfoot. Foot (Edinb) 2020;45:101685.
129. Mengiardi B, Pfirrmann CW, Zanetti M. MR imaging of tendons and ligaments of the midfoot. Semin Musculoskelet Radiol 2005;9(3):187–98.
130. Mengiardi B, Zanetti M, Schöttle PB, et al. Spring ligament complex: MR imaging-anatomic correlation and findings in asymptomatic subjects. Radiology 2005;237(1):242–9.
131. Balen PF, Helms CA. Association of posterior tibial tendon injury with spring ligament injury, sinus tarsi abnormality, and plantar fasciitis on MR imaging. AJR Am J Roentgenol 2001;176(5):1137–43.
132. Deland JT, De Asla RJ, Sung IH, et al. Posterior tibial tendon insufficiency: Which ligaments are involved? Foot Ankle Int 2005;26(6):427–35.
133. Cohen BE, Ogden F. Medial column procedures in the acquired flatfoot deformity. Foot Ankle Clin 2007;12(2):287–99.

Clinical Appearance of Medial Ankle Instability

Roxa Ruiz, MD*, Beat Hintermann, MD

KEYWORDS

- Clinics • Medial ankle instability • First metatarsal rise • Hallux valgus et pronatus
- Foot pronation • Posterior tibial overload • Pseudo hallux rigidus

KEY POINTS

- Medial ankle instability is mainly a clinical diagnosis.
- In an acute injury, tenderness, ecchymosis, and swelling over the deltoid ligament have relatively poor sensitivity.
- In a chronic condition, pain on palpation at anteromedial edge and a valgus and pronation deformity of the loaded foot, which is seen to disappear when the patient is asked to activate the posterior tibial muscle or to go in tiptoe position, are the hallmark for the presence of medial ankle instability.
- Various stress tests permit to identify specific injury patterns of the deltoid and spring ligaments and to elucidate an associated dysfunction of the posterior tibial tendon.
- A hyperactivity of the flexor hallucis longus muscle is typically initiated, which results in an elevation of the first metatarsal head with the appearance of a pseudo hallux rigidus.

INTRODUCTION

Although medial ankle ligament injuries are not rare,[1–4] they are often overlooked, especially in subtle cases, or when overshadowed by lateral ankle injuries.[5] Thus, not surprisingly, the role of medial ligamentous injuries in ankle instability is not well described, similar to the phenomenon of medial ankle instability. Hintermann and colleagues[4] defined several clinical criteria to diagnose medial instability, including the feeling of giving way with pain on the medial gutter of the ankle and a correctable hindfoot valgus and pronation deformity. Based on these criteria, 52 patients were diagnosed with medial ankle instability and treated operatively. Most of the patients (77%) additionally had concomitant lateral ligament injuries, which required repair in 69%. It is thus suggested that medial ankle instability can be present as a result of chronic anterolateral rotational instability or a result of an isolated injury to the superficial deltoid ligament.[6]

Center of Excellence for Foot and Ankle Surgery, Kantonsspital Baselland, Rheinstrasse 26, CH-4410 Liestal, Switzerland
* Corresponding author.
E-mail address: roxa.ruiz@ksbl.ch

Foot Ankle Clin N Am 26 (2021) 291–304
https://doi.org/10.1016/j.fcl.2021.03.004
foot.theclinics.com

The posterior tibial muscle-tendon unit is the main dynamic stabilizer of the hindfoot. The tendon courses behind the medial malleolus under the flexor retinaculum, beyond which it changes direction acutely to insert on the navicular, the cuneiforms, and the bases of the metatarsal bones,[7,8] and this enables the posterior tibial muscle not only to support the medial ligament but also to hide an incompetence of the superficial deltoid ligament.

This result implicates the need to carefully assess the unstable ankle clinically, to be able to diagnose medial ankle instability. The goal of this article is to elucidate the key clinical findings of a medially unstable ankle and to provide the underlying pathologic process that contributes to its clinical appearance. Emphasis is given purely to the ligamentous instability, whereas no focus is given to the deltoid ligament injuries in acute ankle fractures.

HISTORY—INJURY MECHANISM

Acute injuries to the deltoid ligament must be suspected after an eversion and/or pronation injury. Typically, the injury mechanism involves an eversion force applied to the foot while weight bearing, causing a valgus stress to the ankle, or an internal rotation force, causing a pronation stress to the hindfoot. Acute injuries to the deltoid ligament can also occur in association with lateral ankle fractures.

Typically, injuries to the superficial deltoid ligament occur during running down the stairs, landing on uneven surfaces, and dancing while the body simultaneously rotates in the opposite direction. Severe external rotational movements may injure the tibiofibular syndesmotic ligaments in addition.[9] Medial instability should be suspected when patients report a "giving way" feeling, especially toward medial when walking on even ground, down-hill, or downstairs. Patients also report sensing pain at the anteromedial aspect of the ankle and sometimes pain around the lateral ankle, especially during dorsiflexion of the foot.[4,10] Chronic injury may result from overload in patients with an acquired flatfoot deformity.[7,11,12]

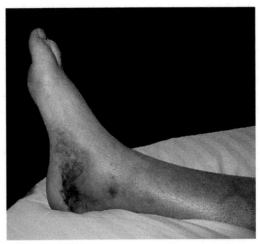

Fig. 1. A 44-year-old female patient with an acute isolated fibular fracture after an external rotation supination trauma. Tenderness, ecchymosis, and swelling seen over the deltoid ligament may indicate an injury to the deltoid ligament; however, it cannot predict the amount of medial ankle instability.

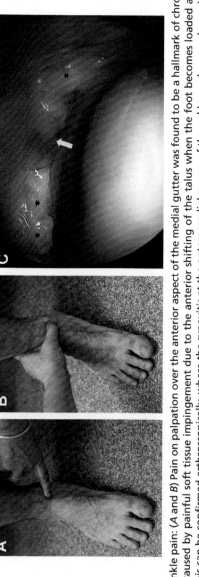

Fig. 2. Medial ankle pain: (*A* and *B*) Pain on palpation over the anterior aspect of the medial gutter was found to be a hallmark of chronic medial ankle instability. It is caused by painful soft tissue impingement due to the anterior shifting of the talus when the foot becomes loaded and/or the foot is pronated. (*C*) This can be confirmed arthroscopically, where the synovitis at the anteromedial corner of the ankle can be seen (*arrow*). Typically, osteophyte formation (*asterix*) can be observed on the anterior rim of the medial tibia and medial malleolus. In most of the cases, superficial cartilage lesions can be seen on the anteromedial talar shoulder as a consequence of the shifting movement.

Injuries to the deep deltoid ligament, in contrast, are mostly seen after a direct eversion trauma, as sustained in contact sports when the foot is enforced in acute eversion by a load applied from lateral to the foot on the ground, for example, when the foot cannot escape.[10]

A direct or indirect trauma that enforces the foot into pronation and abduction may most likely result in an injury to the spring ligament that may include an injury to the posterior tibial tendon at its insertion site[13,14]; this is however not a must. A few studies have reported on adult patients, suffering from an acquired flatfoot deformity caused by isolated spring ligament ruptures, with an intact posterior tibial tendon.[15–19]

An increased risk to injure the deltoid ligament may also be observed in injury mechanisms that involve fractures such as Weber type C/pronation external rotation or pronation abduction and less frequently with Weber B/supination external rotation ankle fractures.[20–24]

CLINICAL FINDINGS

The clinical appearance of medial ankle instability differs between acute and chronic injuries.

Acute Injury

Attempts to use physical examination findings to detect an acute deltoid ligament injury date more than a half century back.[25,26] The conclusions made then have not

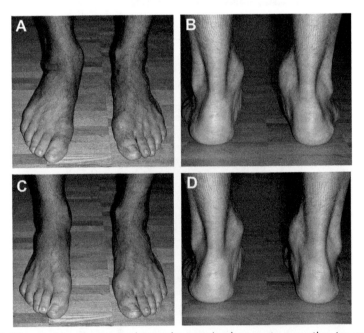

Fig. 3. A 39-year-old male soccer player who sustained an acute pronation trauma of his right ankle 18 months earlier. While weight bearing, the foot takes on a valgus and pronated position. (A) Anterior view. (B) Posterior view. When the patient is asked to activate his posterior tibial muscle, the valgus and pronation deformity is seen to disappear completely. (C) Anterior view. (D) Posterior view.

changed with more recent work.[27–30] Medial tenderness, ecchymosis, and swelling (**Fig. 1**) have relatively poor sensitivity, specificity, and whether positive nor negative predictive value for medial instability (defined as a positive manual external rotation stress test). As a result, physical examination of the medial ankle was essentially abandoned as a modality to assess stability in isolated distal fibula fractures.

Nevertheless, after an acute ankle sprain with or without a fibular fracture, a thorough clinical investigation of the ankle may help diagnose an injury to the deltoid ligament. It should include a careful inspection and palpation to elucidate a hematoma and tenderness and, if possible, an external rotation and eversion stress test.[31] Preoperatively, when the patient is under anesthesia, a stress test under fluoroscopy may help to verify a rupture of the deltoid ligament and quantify the resulting instability.

Chronic Injury

Chronic injuries to the deltoid ligament typically cause medial ankle instability. This instability must be suspected if the patient feels the ankle is about to "give way,"

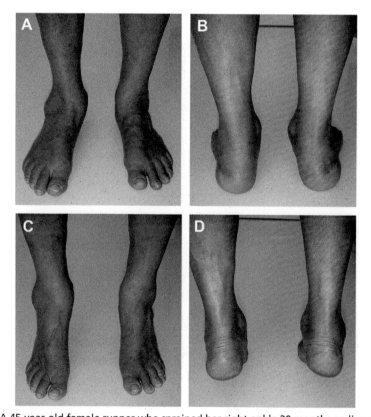

Fig. 4. A 45-year-old female runner who sprained her right ankle 20 months earlier was not specifically treated therefor and is currently suffering from increasing pain and disability. While weight bearing, the foot takes on a valgus and pronated position. (*A*) Anterior view. (*B*) Posterior view. When the patient is asked to go on her tiptoes, the deformity is seen to disappear completely due to the activation of the posterior tibial muscle. (*C*) Anterior view. (*D*) Posterior view.

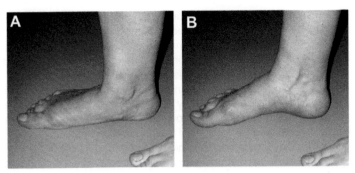

Fig. 5. Preserved function of the posterior tibial tendon can also be seen in this 42-year-old female patient suffering from chronic medial ankle instability. (*A*) When looking at the foot from medial, the weight-bearing foot is pronated and the arch is flattened, whereas the midfoot remains well aligned. (*B*) The foot deformity is fully corrected when the patient is asked to activate the posterior tibial muscle; however, a subtle rise of the first metatarsal can be seen as well as a plantarflexion of the great toe, indicating complementary pull of the flexor hallucis longus tendon to support the function of the posterior tibial muscle.

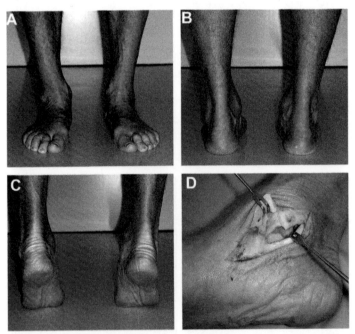

Fig. 6. This 54-year-old male trail runner who sustained a complex sprain of his right ankle 4 years ago is currently suffering from increasing pain that recently also started to be located on the lateral side, not allowing him to run anymore, whereas bicycling is tolerated. While weight bearing, the foot is seen to take on a valgus and pronated position. (*A*) Anterior view. (*B*) Posterior view. When the patient is asked to go on his tiptoes, the deformity is seen to disappear only partially. Notice the remaining medial prominence and the activation of the anterior tibial muscle when trying to correct the deformity. (*C*) Posterior view. (*D*) While radiographically, a talar tilt into valgus of 6° was found (not shown), surgical exploration showed the posterior tibial tendon intact.

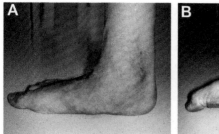
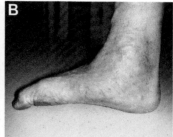

Fig. 7. First metatarsal rise test in a 56-year-old male patient with a posterior tibial tendon dysfunction. (*A*) A picture taken from medial of the weight-bearing right foot, showing a flattened arch and a marked pronation of the hindfoot. (*B*) When the patient is asked to correct the deformity, he cannot keep the first metatarsal on ground; instead, he is seen using the anterior tibial and flexor hallucis longus muscles to correct the hindfoot deformity. The sheath of the posterior tibial tendon is swollen, and no tendon activity can be seen.

especially medially, when walking on even ground, downhill, or downstairs, or if the patient experiences pain at the anteromedial or lateral aspect of the ankle, especially when the foot is dorsiflexed.[4]

A key finding in chronic injuries of the deltoid ligament is pain in the medial gutter, typically provoked by palpation of the anterior border of the medial malleolus (**Fig. 2**).[4,10,32] Such localized pain was found in all 52 patients with medial ankle instability.[4] While weight bearing, increased valgus of the hindfoot and pronation of the affected foot indicate laxity of the medial aspect of the ankle (**Fig. 3**A–B).[4,10,33] Typically, this deformity of the foot is seen to disappear when the patient is asked to activate the posterior tibial muscle (see **Fig. 3**C–D). Analogously, it also disappears when

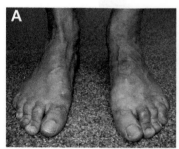
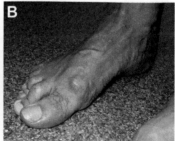
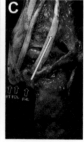

Fig. 8. Pseudo hallux rigidus in a 50-year-old male patient with chronic medial ankle instability in both ankles, however more advanced on the right foot. He was referred to our clinic for treating a hallux rigidus on his right foot. The painful pseudoexostosis is seen on the dorsal aspect of the first metatarsal head, whereas the great toe and the lesser toes are contracted. As a consequence of chronic hyperactivity of the flexor hallucis longus muscle to stabilize the medial ankle, the great toe took on a valgus and pronated position. The anterior tibial muscle is activated on the right side to stabilize the medial arch. (*A*) Anterior view of both feet. (*B*) Medial view of the right foot. (*C*) Anatomic specimen (posterior view) showing the close relationship of posterior tibial tendon with the flexor digitorum longus (FDL) and flexor hallucis longus (FHL) tendons. Notify the action line (*yellow arrow*) of the strong FHL tendon, making this muscle a strong stabilizer of calcaneus against eversion.

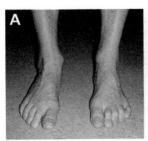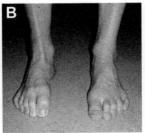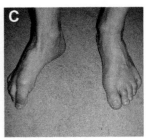

Fig. 9. The compensatory overuse of the flexor hallucis longus muscle to stabilize the medial ankle can be even better seen in this 54-year-old patient who sustained a severe ankle sprain 1.5 years ago. He can pursue his job as a carpenter only with stable high-shaft shoes. Barefoot walking is no longer possible. (*A*) While weight bearing, when compared with the non-affected contralateral side, the foot is seen to be slightly pronated. The deformity is seen to originate at the level of the ankle joint, whereas the foot itself does not show an abduction deformity at the midfoot level. (*B*) When the patient is asked to correct the deformity, besides activating the posterior tibial muscle, he additionally activates the anterior tibial, flexor hallucis longus, and flexor digitorum muscles, thereby supinating the forefoot. (*C*) When trying to walk, the patient uses the plantarflexed great toe to stabilize his ankle.

the patient is asked to go in tiptoe position (**Fig. 4**). The medial arch is also seen to be corrected (**Fig. 5**). With this, a primary posterior tibial tendon dysfunction is excluded. If hindfoot valgus is not fully corrected, it can be due to either a posterior tibial tendon dysfunction or an incompetent deep deltoid (**Fig. 6**). Although pain along the posterior tibial tendon may be present, its inversion force is typically not compromised. The first

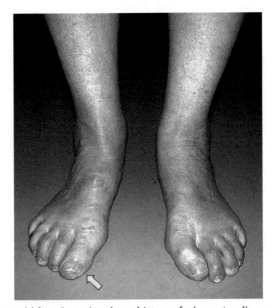

Fig. 10. This 58-year-old female patient has a history of a long-standing medial instability of her right ankle. An extended callosity can be found on the medioplantar aspect of the great toe due to the hyperactivity of the flexor hallucis longus muscle used to stabilize her medial ankle.

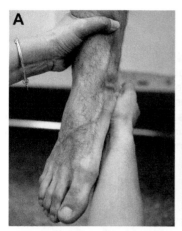
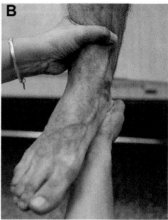

Fig. 11. Eversion stress test. (*A*) With the foot hanging, the distal tibia is held with one hand, whereas the other hand holds the foot at the heel. (*B*) While the foot is in neutral position, the heel is everted and the amount of achieved eversion is compared with the contralateral side.

metatarsal rise sign can also be used to assess posterior tibial function.[34] When the shank is externally rotated or the heel is brought into varus, the first metatarsal head will be elevated if the posterior tibial tendon is dysfunctional. It remains on ground, if normal (**Fig. 7**). All variations of associated flatfoot deformities can be seen if the posterior tibial tendon has subsequently become insufficient. In particular, the forefoot will gradually experience a supination deformity.

In the advanced stage of chronic medial ankle instability, the patient typically presents with a dorsal pseudoexostosis of the first metatarsal head due to an

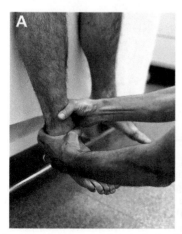
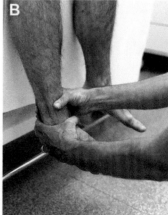

Fig. 12. Anterior drawer test. (*A*) With the foot hanging, the distal tibia is held with one hand, whereas the other hand holds the foot at the heel. (*B*) While the foot is in slight plantar flexion and abduction, the heel is then pulled toward anterior and the anterior translation compared with the contralateral side.

elevated (dorsiflexed) position of the first metatarsal ("Ruiz sign") that may be misinterpreted as a hallux rigidus (**Fig. 8**). When the patient is asked to activate the posterior tibial muscle for correcting the pronation position, the great toe is seen to go into plantarflexion as the patient uses the flexor hallucis longus as a medial ankle stabilizer (**Fig. 9A–B**). When walking barefoot, the patient may even use the plantarflexed great toe to stabilize the foot in the advanced stage (see **Fig. 9C**). Besides this, the great toe typically adapts a valgus and pronated position due to an excessive activation of the flexor hallucis longus muscle to stabilize the medial ankle and medial arch (see **Fig. 8**). Often, a contracture of the lesser toes can also be seen due to a hyperactive flexor digitorum longus muscle (see **Fig. 8**, and **9B**). As a result, a

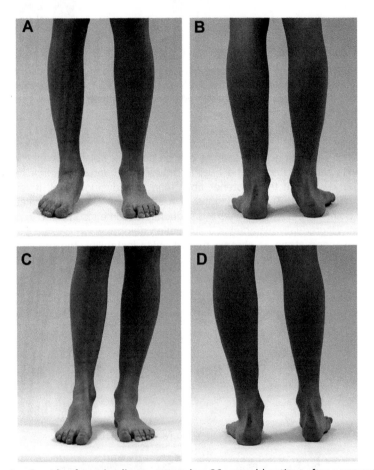

Fig. 13. An example of a spring ligament tear in a 26-year-old patient after a severe trauma by which she landed on the ground with her right foot in a pronated position (neglected for 26 months). (*A*) Anterior view: in addition to a valgus and pronation deformity of the hindfoot, an abduction deformity can be seen at the midfoot level. Notice the valgus and pronation deformity of the great toe as a consequence of a hyperactive flexor hallucis longus muscle, used to stabilize the medial foot. (*B*) The forefoot abduction deformity can be better seen from posterior view. (*C*) Anterior view: the patient is asked to correct the deformity: to do so, she unloads the heel and uses the posterior and anterior tibial muscles to stabilize the ankle. (*D*) The unloading of the heel can be seen better on the posterior view.

callosity formation can be found at the medioplantar aspect of the great toe or at the tip of the lesser toes (**Fig. 10**).

Clinical stress investigation is most reliable when the patient is seated on the table with hanging feet. While the heel is taken with one hand and the tibia with the other hand, a valgus tilt stress is applied to the heel. The result is compared with the contralateral side (**Fig. 11**). Then, while holding the foot in slight plantarflexion and abduction, an anterior drawer stress is applied and again compared with the contralateral side (**Fig. 12**). Anterior dislocation of the talus typically increases when the foot is held in abduction position and decreases when the foot is adducted.

In a chronic condition, it is extremely difficult to clinically test whether the deep deltoid ligament is injured. If the tibiocalcaneal ligament, the strongest part of the superficial deltoid ligament, becomes gradually incompetent, the talus will tilt into valgus and rotate externally, even though the deep deltoid is intact. An isolated incompetence of the deep deltoid ligament, for example, injuries to the anterior and posterior tibiotalar ligaments, is extremely seldom, and it might result in an excessive valgus malalignment of the heel.[32]

Suspicion of a spring ligament injury in isolation should arise clinically, when persistent medial midfoot pain is present with an associated acute pes planus deformity, as typically seen following a trauma with forceful landing on a flatfoot.[16,17] Furthermore, spring ligament deficiency is often present in posterior tibial tendon dysfunction, which results in the adult-acquired pes planus. The clinical presentation is similar to that of an incompetent superficial deltoid ligament, as shown in **Fig. 9**, but it is typically associated with an abduction deformity at the midfoot level (**Fig. 13**). Pasapula and colleagues[35] introduced a clinical examination test to determine the integrity of the spring ligament complex—the neutral heel lateral push test (**Fig. 14**). Experience in using these novel clinical tests to detect various spring ligament injuries still need to be gained to help get a thorough clinical understanding of how they can be used to correctly diagnose medial ankle instability.

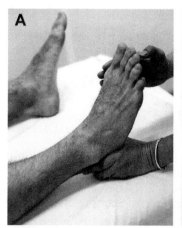
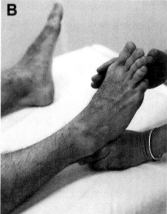

Fig. 14. Heel lateral push test. (*A*) With the foot held in slight dorsiflexed position with one hand at the heel, the forefoot is pushed with the other hand toward laterally. (*B*) With a small force a translation greater than 1 cm can only be attributable to the loss of the integrity of the spring ligament. A translation of 15 to 20 mm can only be achieved when applying firm pressure and when the spring ligament is teared.

SUMMARY

In an acute injury, although the presence of any pain with palpation over the deltoid ligament has a positive correlation with instability, strict reliance on the presence or absence of medial tenderness, ecchymosis, and swelling has relatively poor sensitivity, specificity, and whether positive nor negative predictive value for instability. In a chronic condition, pain on palpation at the anterior aspect of the medial gutter and a valgus and pronation deformity of the loaded foot, which is seen to disappear when the patient is asked to activate the posterior tibial muscle or to go in tiptoe position, are the hallmark for the presence of medial ankle instability. Various stress tests permit to identify specific injury patterns of the deltoid and spring ligaments and to elucidate an associated dysfunction of the posterior tibial tendon. As a defense against the imminent flatfoot deformity, a hyperactivity of the flexor hallucis longus and flexor digitorum longus muscles is typically initiated, which results in changes to the forefoot, such as a contracture of the toes with painful callosity formation and an elevation of the first metatarsal head with the appearance of a pseudo hallux rigidus.

CLINICS CARE POINTS

- Knowledge of the underlying pathology and pathomechanics is mandatory to understand the clinical appearance of medial ankle instability.
- Pain at anteromedial edge of the ankle and a valgus and pronation position that can be actively corrected by asking the patient to activate the posterior tibial muscle or to go in tiptoe position are the hallmark for the presence of medial ankle instability.
- Various stress tests permit to confirm the diagnosis and specify the injury pattern.
- A pseudo hallucis rigidus is the consequence of a hyperactivity of flexor hallucis longus muscle to protect the foot against the valgus and pronation deformity.

DISCLOSURE

The authors declare no potential conflicts of interest with respect to the research, authorship, and/or publication of this article.

REFERENCES

1. Alshalawi S, Galhoum AE, Alrashidi Y, et al. Medial ankle instability: the deltoid dilemma. Foot Ankle Clin 2018;23(4):639–57.
2. Crim J. Medial-sided ankle pain: deltoid ligament and beyond. Magn Reson Imaging Clin N Am 2017;25(1):63–77.
3. Hintermann B, Boss A, Schafer D. Arthroscopic findings in patients with chronic ankle instability. Am J Sports Med 2002;30(3):402–9.
4. Hintermann B, Valderrabano V, Boss A, et al. Medial ankle instability: an exploratory, prospective study of fifty-two cases. Am J Sports Med 2004;32(1):183–90.
5. Crim JR, Beals TC, Nickisch F, et al. Deltoid ligament abnormalities in chronic lateral ankle instability. Foot Ankle Int 2011;32(9):873–8.
6. Hintermann B. Biomechanics of the unstable ankle joint and clinical implications. Med Sci Sports Exerc 1999;31(7 Suppl):S459–69.
7. Deland JT, de Asla RJ, Sung IH, et al. Posterior tibial tendon insufficiency: which ligaments are involved? Foot Ankle Int 2005;26(6):427–35.

8. Hintermann B. Biomechanical aspects of muscle-tendon functions. Orthopade 1995;24(3):187–92.

9. Massri-Pugin J, Lubberts B, Vopat BG, et al. Role of the deltoid ligament in syndesmotic instability. Foot Ankle Int 2018;39(5):598–603.

10. Hintermann B. Medial ankle instability. Foot Ankle Clin 2003;8(4):723–38.

11. Kitaoka HB, Luo ZP, An KN. Reconstruction operations for acquired flatfoot: biomechanical evaluation. Foot Ankle Int 1998;19(4):203–7.

12. Hintermann B, Valderrabano V, Kundert HP. Lengthening of the lateral column and reconstruction of the medial soft tissue for treatment of acquired flatfoot deformity associated with insufficiency of the posterior tibial tendon. Foot Ankle Int 1999;20(10):622–9.

13. Masaragian HJ, Massetti S, Perin F, et al. Flatfoot deformity due to isolated spring ligament injury. J Foot Ankle Surg 2020;59(3):469–78.

14. Hintermann B, Ruiz R. Medial ankle instability (including Spring ligament). In: Hintermann B, Ruiz R, editors. Foot and Ankle Instability. A Clinical Guide to Diagnosis and Surgical Management. Springer; 2021.

15. Masaragian HJ, Ricchetti HO, Testa C. Acute isolated rupture of the spring ligament: a case report and review of the literature. Foot Ankle Int 2013;34(1):150–4.

16. Borton DC, Saxby TS. Tear of the plantar calcaneonavicular (spring) ligament causing flatfoot. A case report. J Bone Joint Surg Br 1997;79(4):641–3.

17. Orr JD, Nunley JA 2nd. Isolated spring ligament failure as a cause of adult-acquired flatfoot deformity. Foot Ankle Int 2013;34(6):818–23.

18. Shuen V, Prem H. Acquired unilateral pes planus in a child caused by a ruptured plantar calcaneonavicular (spring) ligament. J Pediatr Orthop B 2009;18(3):129–30.

19. Williams G, Widnall J, Evans P, et al. Could failure of the spring ligament complex be the driving force behind the development of the adult flatfoot deformity? J Foot Ankle Surg 2014;53(2):152–5.

20. Butler BA, Hempen EC, Barbosa M, et al. Deltoid ligament repair reduces and stabilizes the talus in unstable ankle fractures. J Orthop 2020;17:87–90.

21. Lee S, Lin J, Hamid KS, et al. Deltoid ligament rupture in ankle fracture: diagnosis and management. J Am Acad Orthop Surg 2019;27(14):e648–58.

22. Gougoulias N, Sakellariou A. When is a simple fracture of the lateral malleolus not so simple? how to assess stability, which ones to fix and the role of the deltoid ligament. The bone Jt J 2017;99-B(7):851–5.

23. van den Bekerom MP, Mutsaerts EL, van Dijk CN. Evaluation of the integrity of the deltoid ligament in supination external rotation ankle fractures: a systematic review of the literature. Arch Orthop Trauma Surg 2009;129(2):227–35.

24. Stufkens SA, van den Bekerom MP, Knupp M, et al. The diagnosis and treatment of deltoid ligament lesions in supination-external rotation ankle fractures: a review. Strateg Trauma Limb Reconstr 2012;7(2):73–85.

25. Cedell CA. Supination-outward rotation injuries of the ankle. A clinical and roentgenological study with special reference to the operative treatment. Acta Orthop Scand 1967;(Suppl 110):113.

26. Lauge-Hansen N. Ligamentous ankle fractures; diagnosis and treatment. Acta Chir Scand 1949;97(6):544–50.

27. Egol KA, Amirtharajah M, Tejwani NC, et al. Ankle stress test for predicting the need for surgical fixation of isolated fibular fractures. J Bone Joint Surg Am 2004;86(11):2393–8.

28. DeAngelis NA, Eskander MS, French BG. Does medial tenderness predict deep deltoid ligament incompetence in supination-external rotation type ankle fractures? J Orthop Trauma 2007;21(4):244–7.

29. McConnell T, Creevy W, Tornetta P 3rd. Stress examination of supination external rotation-type fibular fractures. J Bone Joint Surg Am 2004;86(10):2171–8.

30. Stenquist DS, Miller C, Velasco B, et al. Medial tenderness revisited: is medial ankle tenderness predictive of instability in isolated lateral malleolus fractures? Injury 2020;51(6):1392–6.

31. Gibson PD, Ippolito JA, Hwang JS, et al. Physiologic widening of the medial clear space: What's normal? J Clin Orthop Trauma 2019;10(Suppl 1):S62–4.

32. Hintermann B, Knupp M, Pagenstert GI. Deltoid ligament injuries: diagnosis and management. Foot Ankle Clin 2006;11(3):625–37.

33. Nelson DR, Younger A. Acute posttraumatic planovalgus foot deformity involving hindfoot ligamentous pathology. Foot Ankle Clin 2003;8(3):521–37.

34. Hintermann B, Gachter A. The first metatarsal rise sign: a simple, sensitive sign of tibialis posterior tendon dysfunction. Foot Ankle Int 1996;17(4):236–41.

35. Pasapula C, Devany A, Magan A, et al. Neutral heel lateral push test: the first clinical examination of spring ligament integrity. Foot (Edinb) 2015;25(2):69–74.

Arthroscopic Assessment and Treatment of Medial Collateral Ligament Complex

Jordi Vega, MD[a,b,c],*, Matteo Guelfi, MD[d,e,f]

KEYWORDS

- Ankle instability • Medial ankle instability • Medial collateral ligament
- Rotational ankle instability • Ankle arthroscopy • Ligament repair

KEY POINTS

- Injury of the medial collateral ligament (MCL) complex can result in medial ankle instability (MAI) or rotational ankle instability (RAI).
- An injury of the anterior fibers of the MCL secondary to an ATFL insufficiency is possible, and this pattern has been defined as RAI; whereas, injury of the intermediate fibers of the MCL will result in an MAI.
- Chronic ankle instability may present concomitant intraarticular pathologies, and this may cause postoperative symptoms when not treated. Because these conditions can often not be detected on imaging studies, arthroscopy has evolved as a helpful and important diagnostic tool, and it enables the surgeon to define the best treatment strategy.
- Repair of MCL injury by an arthroscopic all-inside procedure is an effectiveness technique when treating either MAI or RAI.

INTRODUCTION

The medial collateral ligament (MCL) complex can be affected by different pathologic conditions.

MCL acute or chronic injuries are usually a result of an ankle sprain or chronic overload, as the case of a long-standing posterior tibialis dysfunction.[1]

Acute MCL injuries usually involve pronation external rotation or less common supination external rotation sprains.[2] According to the trauma mechanism, the sprain may

[a] Human Anatomy and Embryology Unit, Department of Pathology and Experimental Therapeutics, University of Barcelona, Barcelona, Spain; [b] MIFAS (Minimally Invasive Foot and Ankle Society) by GRECMIP (Groupe de Recherche et d'Étude en Chirurgie Mini-Invasive du Pied), Merignac, France; [c] Foot and Ankle Unit, Orthopedic Department, iMove Tres Torres, Barcelona, Spain; [d] Casa di Cura Villa Montallegro, Via Monte Zovetto 27, Genoa 16145, Italy; [e] Department of Orthopaedic Surgery "Gruppo Policlinico di Monza", Clinica Salus, Alessandria, Italy; [f] Human Anatomy and Embryology Unit, Department of Morphological Sciences, Universitat Autònoma de Barcelona, Barcelona, Spain
* Corresponding author. iMove Tres Torres, Barcelona 08017, Spain.
E-mail address: jordivega@hotmail.com

Foot Ankle Clin N Am 26 (2021) 305–313
https://doi.org/10.1016/j.fcl.2021.03.005
foot.theclinics.com

lead to lateral and/or medial malleolus fracture, syndesmosis injury, or MCL injury. Isolated MCL injuries, however, are rarely observed.[3,4] In these cases, acute surgical repair of MCL injury is controversial, and usually a conservative therapy is proposed.[5,6] When conservative therapy fails, patient can develop a medial ankle instability (MAI).[7,8] MAI is defined as a medial giving way when walking or during sports, and typically an asymmetric hindfoot valgus can be seen in relaxed position while weight bearing.

Ankle sprains are a common injury.[9] Ankle inversion is the most common mechanism of injury, and it typically results in a lesion of lateral ligaments. After an acute ankle inversion sprain, between 15% and 20% of patients will develop a chronic ankle instability (CAI), and they will experience repetitive ankle sprains.[10] In CAI an incompetent anterior talofibular ligament (ATFL) cause an increased anterolateral extrusion of talus out of the mortise, talar internal rotation, and superior translation.[11] These biomechanical changes may cause several intraarticular pathologies and degenerative arthritis. Injury of MCL has been observed in as much as 40% of patients with CAI.[12,13] Recently, a new concept of ankle instability named rotational ankle instability (RAI) has been described.[14,15] RAI is defined as an abnormal talar rotation within the tibiofibular mortise, with subsequently increased internal talar rotation, which may stretch out the superficial deltoid ligament that have become overloaded.[14]

In the last 2 decades, ankle arthroscopy has significant evolved and new arthroscopic techniques have been developed to treat ankle ligaments injury.[16] The usefulness of arthroscopy has been established for both the acute[14] and, even more, the chronic MCL injury. Arthroscopic ligament repair has also been recently described to treat MCL injury with excellent results.[14]

The aim of this article is to highlight the role of ankle arthroscopy in diagnosis and treatment of MAI and RAI. In addition, an arthroscopic description of MCL intraarticular anatomy and an arthroscopic classification of MCL injury are proposed.

CLINICAL PRESENTATION

Patients with both MAI and RAI may report on a history of ankle sprain. Because the underlying pathology involving the MCL is different between these 2 entities, they are discussed separately through the manuscript.

Isolated MAI is a rare presentation. Patients with CAI may have a predisposition to MCL injury, such as flatfoot deformity, hyper-pronation, or laxity.[12,13] Patients with MAI may indicate medial and lateral ankle symptoms such as pain, swelling, and tenderness, or a combination of them. Several physical tests ranging from talar tilt test, valgus test, or external rotation test have been proposed to evaluate mechanical competence of the MCL.[7,17,18] However, frequently no signs are observed in most patients, and these physical tests have been reported inadequate when evaluating MAI.[19] An asymmetric hindfoot valgus and pronation deformity can be typically seen with weight bearing, whereas the patient is usually able to correct the deformity when asked to activate the posterior tibial muscle.

RAI is difficult to assess clinically. It is estimated that 10% to 15% of patients with CAI will develop an RAI, although in authors' experience this percentage may be underestimated.[14] Patients with RAI report chronic symptoms of lateral ankle instability and medial ankle pain and tenderness located at the anterior area of the medial malleolus. Medial symptoms usually are reported often later than the lateral ankle instability appeared. As much as 23% of patients, however, were found to never report medial ankle symptoms, and thus the MAI remains neglected.[14]

In every patient who has sustained an ankle sprain, the medial side of the ankle should therefore be carefully investigated for pain, tenderness, and ligament incompetence with subsequent valgus and pronation deformity. When a restrain deficit of the most anterior facet of the deltoid ligament exists, the talus can anteriorly translate and subsequently externally rotate within the ankle mortise, which may result in a medial rotational instability.

ARTHROSCOPIC ASSESSMENT

Ankle arthroscopy is performed in a supine position and under tourniquet. Usually, two standard ankle arthroscopic portals are used, anteromedial and anterolateral. The anteromedial portal is created first and placed at the ankle joint line just medial to the tibialis anterior tendon. The anterolateral portal is placed just lateral to the peroneus tertius tendon or to the extensor digitorum longus tendons, paying attention not to injure the intermediate dorsocutaneous nerve, a branch of the superficial peroneal nerve.

The arthroscope is first introduced through the anteromedial portal. It is recommended to use a protocolized arthroscopic evaluation of the ankle joint in order to detect all possible intraarticular pathologies. Arthroscopic examination of the anterior ankle compartment includes seven points[20]: (1) anterior tibiofibular ligament (ATiFL's) distal fascicle; (2) ATFL's superior fascicle (lateral gutter); (3) lateral talar neck; (4) medial talar neck; (5) deep layer of MCL and tip of the medial malleolus (medial gutter); (6) medial tibial angle (notch of Henry); and (7) anterior tibial rim. The arthroscope may be switched to the anteromedial portal to better visualize the medial ankle compartment.[21] Most importantly, arthroscopic assessment of lateral and medial gutters should be performed in a slightly dorsiflexed position and without distraction, which allows full visualization of lateral and medial gutters and evaluation of intraarticular ligaments.[20] Intraarticular ligaments include the ATFL's superior fascicle and the ATiFL's distal fascicle at the anterolateral side and the MCL's deep fascicles at the medial side.[20]

Intraarticular fatty tissue generally occupies the central and medial aspect of the anterior ankle compartment; it may be resected with shaver to allow for full arthroscopic visualization of the medial malleolus and the MCL. In particular, the surgeon should be aware that the medial malleolus is covered by a thin fringe of cartilage that articulates with the medial wall of the talus, next a central fringe of cortical bone and the insertion of the deep MCL fascicles. In dorsiflexion, the deep MCL fascicles can be seen on the bottom of the medial gutter as a hammocklike structure between the medial wall of the talus and the medial malleolus. The anterior fascicles, the tibiotalar and tibionavicular ligament, are attached to the anterior aspect of the anterior colliculus of the medial malleolus, whereas intermediate fascicles, the tibiospring and tibiocalcaneal ligament, are attached to the tip of anterior colliculus of the medial malleolus. The MCL posterior fascicle, composed by the posterior tibiotalar ligament, is not visible by anterior arthroscopy.

These anatomic features are crucial for MCL injury recognition. Any arthroscopic vision that differs from the normally described on the medial gutter should raise the suspicion of MCL tear. When an injury of MCL is suspected, the examination should be completed with the arthroscope introduced through the anterolateral portal and the probe through the anteromedial portal (**Fig. 1**).

An arthroscopic classification for unstable ankles based on the widening of the tibiotalar joint space was proposed by Hintermann and colleagues.[7] A more or less difficult instruments that pass through the tibiotalar space allowed the surgeon to grade the instability. This classification graded the ankle joint as follows: stable, when some

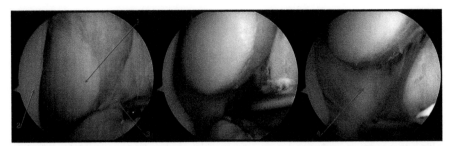

Fig. 1. Arthroscopic exploration of the medial collateral ligament (right ankle). The scope is introduced through the anterolateral portal. The anterior and intermediate fascicles of the deep layer of medial collateral ligament are examined with the help of the probe or shaver. (1) Medial malleolus; (2) medial talar wall; (3) anterior fascicle of the medial collateral ligament; (4) intermediate fascicle of the medial collateral ligament.

translocation of the talus is present but not enough to introduce the 5 mm arthroscope into the tibiotalar space; moderately unstable, when the tibiotalar joint space is wide enough to introduce a 5 mm arthroscope, but not more than 5 mm; severely unstable, when the talus is moved easily out of the ankle mortise, which typically allows for free insight into the posterior aspect of the ankle joint. In the same study, a specific classification of medial instability by open surgery has been proposed. This divided medial instability into proximal, intermediate, and distal injuries of the MCL. To the authors' knowledge an arthroscopic classification of MAI is missing in literature.

Arthroscopic Classification of Medial Collateral Ligament Injury

Based on arthroscopic findings, MCL injury can be divided into injury of the MCL anterior fascicle (tibiotalar and tibionavicular ligaments) or the MCL intermediate fascicle (tibiospring and tibiocalcaneal ligaments) (**Table 1**).

Injury affecting the anterior fascicle is described as the open book lesion, and it describes an RAI.[12] Open book injury is only observed when talar internal rotation or the instruments push the ligament to medial. Then, the MCL anterior fascicle is observed separated from the medial malleolus. Open book can be graded into 2 types according to instruments that pass through the space between the medial malleolus and the MCL anterior fascicle (**Fig. 2**):

Table 1 Arthroscopic classification of medial collateral ligament injury			
Tear Location	**Instability**	**Grade**	**Description**
Anterior fibers of deltoid ligament (tibiotalar and tibionavicular ligament)	RAI—the MCL injury is secondary to a partial or complete injury of the LCL (see **Fig. 2**)	Type 1	Open book injury with instruments not allowed to pass through
		Type 2	Open book injury with instruments allowed to pass through
Intermediate fibers of deltoid ligament (tibiospring and tibiocalcaneal ligament)	MAI—the MCL injury could be either isolated or associated to an LCL injury (see **Fig. 3**)	Type 1	Partial injury (wave shape)
		Type 2	Complete injury

Abbreviation: LCL, lateral collateral ligament.

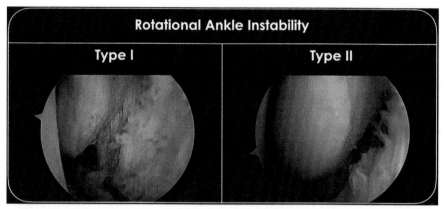

Fig. 2. Types of medial collateral ligament open book injury in rotational ankle instability. In type I, instruments are not allowed to pass through between the ligament and the medial malleolus. When type II injury is observed, instruments are allowed to pass through between the ligament and the medial malleolus.

Type 1: open book injury with instruments not allowed to pass through.

Type 2: open book injury with instruments allowed to pass through.

Injury affecting the MCL intermediate fascicle is observed in patients with MAI. Because the deep MCL fascicles are shorter than that from the superficial fascicles, deep MCL fascicles are more prone to injury after an eversion ankle trauma. Although the MCL deep fascicle can probably be injured along its length, the ligament injury has always been arthroscopically observed at the level of the medial malleolus attachment (in its anterior colliculus) and never at midportion or talar attachment (**Fig. 3**):

Type 1: partial injury or wave shape injury.

Type 2: complete injury.

ARTHROSCOPIC TREATMENT

The role of arthroscopy in treatment of ankle instability has increased during last years. Given the success of arthroscopic lateral ankle ligament repair or reconstruction,[16,22,23]

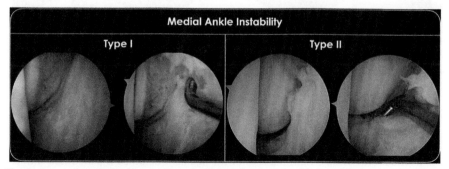

Fig. 3. Types of medial collateral ligament injury in medial ankle instability. Type I is characterized by a partial injury (wave shape) of the intermediate fascicle of the medial collateral ligament, whereas type II is characterized by a complete injury of the intermediate fascicle of the medial collateral ligament.

some investigators have evolved techniques for repairing the MCL by arthroscopic technique to decrease the recovery time postoperatively and facilitate an earlier return to full function.[14,24,25]

After having completed the arthroscopic examination, the concomitant intraarticular pathologies, if present, will be addressed arthroscopically. Thereafter, the MCL tear is treated.

An arthroscopic-assisted technique of treating MCL tear has been described by 2 different investigators.[24,25] The suture anchors are introduced through the arthroscopic portals, and the sutures are passed percutaneously through the ligament. It has been described as a safe procedure.[24]

The arthroscopic all-inside repair of the MCL with a knotless suture-anchor technique was the first described arthroscopic all-inside method of treating MCL tear and without any percutaneous step.[14] With this procedure, repair is made to the MCL under direct arthroscopic view and through an all-inside technique (**Figs. 4** and **5**). Although excellent preliminary results with low rates of minor complications have been reported to treat RAI,[14] it can also be used to treat MAI. To the author's experience, the arthroscopic all-inside MCL repair yields excellent results treating both RAI and MAI.

In the cases with an associated injury of the lateral collateral ligament, it should be treated after completing the MCL repair in order to not stress the ligament repair during flexion and extension of the ankle. The arthroscopic all-inside repair technique as previously reported is the technique of choice.[26–28]

As a general postoperative protocol, a removable walker boot is maintained for 3 to 4 weeks postoperative at all times. Weight bearing as tolerated with the aid of crutches is encouraged. In cases of chondral or osteochondral injuries, no weight bearing is allowed for 4 to 6 weeks. Antithrombotic prophylaxis is indicated minimally for the first 15 days postoperative. Once the walking boot is removed, active and passive range of motion exercises and gait training are encouraged. Two weeks later, strengthening in ankle dorsiflexion, plantarflexion, eversion, and inversion, as well as proprioceptive training with weight bearing are initiated. Noncontact sports (swimming or cycling) are allowed 2 months postoperatively, and unrestricted sports, including contact sports, can be expected at 3 months depending on muscle conditioning.

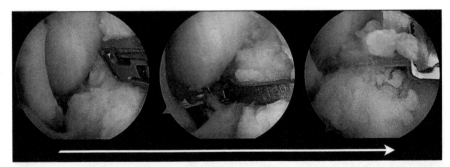

Fig. 4. Under arthroscopic view, the area of the ligament detached is penetrated with an automatic suture passer clamp introduced through the anteromedial portal. Once the ligament is penetrated by a double high resistance suture, one or both ends of the suture are introduced into the suture loop, and by pulling the ends, the loop is introduced into the joint and the ligament is grasped.

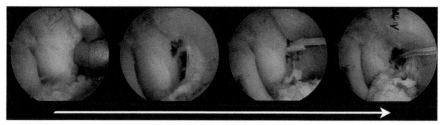

Fig. 5. The tunnel for the bone anchor is drilled on the anterior aspect of the medial malleolus. Finally, the medial collateral ligament is reattached to the medial malleolus with a knotless bone anchor.

RESULTS

To the authors' knowledge, only a few studies are available in the literature reporting on arthroscopic treatment of MCL injury.[14,24] Recently, an arthroscopic-assisted MCL repair associated to a percutaneous passage reported a 90% satisfaction rate in a group of 87 patients.[24] Of these, the MCL injury was not associated to an ankle fracture in only 30 patients. Despite a high satisfaction rate, 6 of 30 patients with MAI reported a persistent ankle pain at final follow-up.

The authors reported previously on combined arthroscopic all-inside repair of both lateral and medial ankle ligaments in 13 patients with the diagnosis of RAI.[14] At the time of follow-up, all patients reported subjective improvement in ankle stability and returned to their daily activities without difficulties, except one patient who continued to experience medial ankle pain. Patients who had engaged in sports returned to their preinjury activity without limitations. The median American Orthopaedic Foot and Ankle Society (AOFAS) score increased from 70 (range 44–77) preoperatively to 100 (range 77–100) at the time of final follow-up. In all patients, the anterior drawer test and talar tilt were negative on clinical examination. Five patients (38.5%) experienced ankle plantarflexion deficit compared with the contralateral side; the deficit was less than 10° in all cases. Two patients (15.4%) had a deficit of 5° or less in ankle dorsiflexion, reporting mild discomfort when squatting or kneeling. Deficit in range of motion was not considered a complication but as a consequence of the arthroscopic ankle stabilization. No major complications were reported.

SUMMARY

In the last years, ankle arthroscopy has contributed to a better understanding of ankle instability, especially regarding MCL injury, and new treatment concepts by arthroscopy were developed. Two different types of MCL injury can be observed, MAI and RAI. MAI as a result of injury of the intermediate MCL fascicles may occur isolated or combined to lateral CAI. When there is RAI, injury of the anterior MCL fascicles is secondary to an insufficiency of the lateral collateral ligament.

Because ankle instability is often associated to intraarticular pathologies that may generate pain and dysfunction, arthroscopy plays an important role in identifying and treating all intraarticular abnormalities besides ligament repair. It is suggested that treatment of associated abnormalities may provide better clinical outcomes.

Despite a few studies are available in literature on arthroscopic treatment of MCL injury, arthroscopic all-inside repair of lateral and medial ankle ligaments has shown evidence of providing promising clinical results. However, further clinical studies are needed to evaluate the clinical outcomes of arthroscopic treatment of MCL injury.

DISCLOSURE

The authors have nothing to disclose.

REFERENCES

1. Deland JT, de Asla RJ, Sung IH, et al. Posterior tibial tendon insufficiency: which ligaments are involved? Foot Ankle Int 2005;26(6):427–35.
2. Lauge-Hansen N. Fractures of the ankle. III. Genetic roentgenologic diagnosis of fractures of the ankle. Am J Roentgenol Radium Ther Nucl Med 1954;71(3): 456–71.
3. Ribbans WJ, Garde A. Tibialis posterior tendon and deltoid and spring ligament injuries in the elite athlete. Foot Ankle Clin 2013;18(2):255–91.
4. Gerber JP, Williams GN, Scoville CR, et al. Persistent disability associated with ankle sprains: a prospective examination of an athletic population. Foot Ankle Int 1998;19(10):653–60.
5. Lee TH, Jang KS, Choi GW, et al. The contribution of anterior deltoid ligament to ankle stability in isolated lateral malleolar fractures. Injury 2016;47(7):1581–5.
6. Strömsöe K, Höqevold HE, Skjeldal S, et al. The repair of a ruptured deltoid ligament is not necessary in ankle fractures. J Bone Joint Surg Br 1995;77(6):920–1.
7. Hintermann B. Medial ankle instability. Foot Ankle Clin 2003;8(4):723–38.
8. Knupp M, Horn Lang T, Zwicky L, et al. Chronic ankle instability (medial and lateral). Clin Sports Med 2015;34(4):679–88.
9. Ferran NA, Maffulli N. Epidemiology of sprains of the lateral ankle ligament complex. Foot Ankle Clin 2006;11:659–62.
10. DiGiovanni BF, Partal G, Baumhauer JF. Acute ankle injury and chronic lateral instability in the athlete. Clin Sports Med 2004;23(1):1–19.
11. Caputo AM, Lee JY, Spritzer CE, et al. In vivo kinematics of the tibiotalar joint after lateral ankle instability. Am J Sports Med 2009;37(11):2241–8.
12. Hintermann B, Boss A, Schäfer D. Arthroscopic findings in patients with chronic ankle instability. Am J Sports Med 2002;30(3):402–9.
13. Schäfer D, Hintermann B. Arthroscopic assessment of the chronic unstable ankle joint. Knee Surg Sports Traumatol Arthrosc 1996;4(1):48–52.
14. Vega J, Allmendinger J, Malagelada F, et al. Combined arthroscopic all-inside repair of lateral and medial ankle ligaments is an effective treatment for rotational ankle instability. Knee Surg Sports Traumatol Arthrosc 2020;28(1):132–40.
15. Buchhorn T, Sabeti-Aschraf M, Dlaska CE, et al. Combined medial and lateral anatomic ligament reconstruction for chronic rotational instability of the ankle. Foot Ankle Int 2011;32(12):1122–6.
16. Vega J, Dalmau-Pastor M, Malagelada F, et al. Ankle arthroscopy: an update. J Bone Joint Surg Am 2017;99(16):1395–407.
17. Richardson DR. Ankle injuries. In: Canale ST, Beaty JH, editors. Campbell's operative orthopaedics. 11th edition. Philadelphia: Mosby Elsevier; 2007. p. 2353–89.
18. Beals TC, Crim J, Nickisch F. Deltoid ligament injuries in athletes: techniques of repair and reconstruction. Oper Tech Sports Med 2010;18(1):11–7.
19. Van den Bekerom MP, Mutsaerts EL, Van Dijk CN. Evaluation of the integrity of the deltoid ligament in supination external rotation ankle fractures: a systematic review of the literature. Arch Orthop Trauma Surg 2009;129(2):227–35.
20. Dalmau-Pastor M, Malagelada F, Kerkhoffs GMMJ, et al. Redefining anterior ankle arthroscopic anatomy: medial and lateral ankle collateral ligaments are visible through dorsiflexion and non-distraction anterior ankle arthroscopy. Knee Surg Sports Traumatol Arthrosc 2020;28(1):18–23.

21. Vega J, Malagelada F, Kerkhoffs GMMJ, et al. A step - by - step arthroscopic examination of the anterior ankle compartment. Knee Surg Sports Traumatol Arthrosc 2020;28(1):24–33.

22. Acevedo JI, Palmer RC, Mangone PG. Arthroscopic treatment of ankle instability: Brostrom. Foot Ankle Clin 2018;23(4):555–70.

23. Glazebrook M, Eid M, Alhadhoud M, et al. Percutaneous Ankle Reconstruction of Lateral Ligaments. Foot Ankle Clin 2018;23(4):581–92.

24. Acevedo JI, Kreulen C, Cedeno AA, et al. Technique for arthroscopic deltoid ligament repair with description of safe zones. Foot Ankle Int 2020;41(5):605–11.

25. Kim JG, Gwak HC, Lee MJ, et al. Arthroscopic deltoid repair: A technical tip. J Foot Ankle Surg 2017;56(6):1253–6.

26. Vega J, Guelfi M, Heyrani N, et al. Ankle microinstability. Tech Foot Ankle Surg 2019;18(2):73–9.

27. Vega J, Golanó P, Pellegrino A, et al. All-inside arthroscopic lateral collateral ligament repair for ankle instability with a knotless suture anchor technique. Foot Ankle Int 2013;34(12):1701–9.

28. Vega J, Guelfi M, Malagelada F, et al. Arthroscopic all-Inside anterior talofibular ligament repair through a three-portal and no-ankle-distraction technique. JBJS Essent Surg Tech 2018;8(3):1–11.

Current Concepts in Treatment of Acute Deltoid Instability

Gastón Slullitel, MD*, Juan Pablo Calvi, MD

KEYWORDS

- Deltoid ligament • Medial instability • Medial collateral ligament • Acute treatment

KEY POINTS

- Isolated deltoid ligament injury accounts for 5% of all ankle ligament injuries.
- There is a large void in the literature when assessing the isolated deltoid sprain in the acute setting.
- The misdiagnosis of acute deltoid ligament injury could ultimately result in chronic medial ankle instability.
- Stable lesions are best treated conservatively, yet the optimal treatment of unstable lesions is controversial.

CRITICAL TREATMENT HIGHLIGHTS

- Medial ankle sprains have been reported to result in significantly greater time lost and long-term disability than lateral ankle ligament injuries.
- The paramount aspect of adequate diagnosis of acute deltoid ligament injury is to determine whether the lesion is stable or unstable.
- Pain and ecchymosis usually reflect ligament injury, but they are not reliable for determining instability.
- MRI ability to detect injury to any portion of the deltoid complex reported a sensitivity of 84% and a specificity of 93%.
- Ultrasonography can discriminate the injured deltoid layers and the site of the injury and allows the performance of dynamic maneuvers.
- Ruling out previous medial or lateral instability and addressing the foot type are important in defining surgical versus conservative treatment.

Foot and Ankle Surgery Department, J Slullitel Institute of Orthopaedics, San Luis 2534, Rosario, Santa Fe 2000, Argentina
* Corresponding author.
E-mail address: gastonslullitel@gmail.com
Twitter: @gatoslullitel (G.S.); @pieijs (J.P.C.)

Foot Ankle Clin N Am 26 (2021) 315–327
https://doi.org/10.1016/j.fcl.2021.03.006
foot.theclinics.com

BACKGROUND

In only 5% of ankle sprains, the deltoid ligament is solely involved.[1] Deltoid ligament injuries may occur either as a consequence of protonation or supination, external rotation mechanism.[2,3] Medial ankle sprains have been reported to result in significantly greater time lost and long-term disability.[1,4]

Signs and symptoms that are usually associated with acute deltoid ligament injury include medial ecchymosis, tenderness, and swelling, and in more severe lesions radiographic manifestations of instability (medial clear space widening and lateral talar shifting, and/or medial talar tilt).[5] However, even in the scenario of an eversion sprain, those symptoms may be so tenuous that they are missed without appropriate examination. Neglecting a deltoid ligament injury may ultimately result in chronic medial ankle instability, which may lead to disability and eventually to ankle osteoarthritis.[5] A validated prognostic factor of progression to ankle arthritis (eg, amount of widening, valgus tilt, foot type) has not yet been defined. However, it has been discussed that even without widening of the medial clear space, valgus tilt can occur if there is a complete deltoid tear, and that could be the factor that leads to progression of the disability and ultimately arthritis.

When analyzing acute deltoid instability without bony injury, three different scenarios may be considered: (1) an isolated deltoid lesion, (2) an injury to the deltoid in the setting of a rotational ankle instability, and (3) an injury to the deltoid ligament associated to a syndesmotic (distal tibiofibular) ligament injury.

Although thoroughly discussed in the context of an ankle fracture or even in the rotational sprain, there is a large void in the literature when assessing the isolated deltoid sprain in the acute setting.

This article thoroughly discusses the isolated acute deltoid ligament impairment, and succinctly analyzes the other two scenarios because they are topics of further articles.

PATHOPHYSIOLOGY

The deltoid ligament shows a complex ligament structure spanning from the medial malleolus of the ankle to the navicular, talus, and calcaneus bones.[6] The superficial layers of the deltoid ligament specifically limit talar abduction or negative talar tilt. The talocalcaneal ligament specifically limits talar protonation, whereas the deep layers of the deltoid ligament restrain medial talar tilt and external rotation. Depending on the mechanism of injury, different fascicles may be involved.

Deltoid ligament injuries can occur while running downstairs, landing on an uneven surface, and dancing with the body simultaneously rotating in the opposite direction, thus sustaining a protonation (eversion) trauma (eg, an outward rotation of the foot during simultaneous inward rotation of the tibia).[2,7,8] Excessive lateral rotation may injure the tibiofibular and interosseous ligaments at the syndesmosis. The anterior fibers of the deltoid ligament may also be involved in extreme rotation injuries.[2] Typically, the foot is firm on the ground when an eversion force causes a valgus stress to the ankle, or an internal rotation force causes a protonation stress to the hindfoot.[2] Acute injuries to the deltoid ligament frequently occur in association with lateral ankle fracture. Complete acute rupture of the deltoid ligament can also be seen in athletes after a valgus trauma, without injury to the lateral aspect of the ankle.[9]

Disruption of the medial deltoid ligament complex allows the talus to tilt within the mortise and/or to laterally migrate if the syndesmotic ligaments are also involved. Another possible scenario for talar tilt is combined medial and lateral ligament disruption in the absence of syndesmotic injury. This is a frequent situation in the setting of a moderate to severe medial sprain in which rotational forces were involved. Such misalignment results in altered joint mechanics. Studies have shown that even small deviations from anatomic alignment result in a greatly reduced joint contact area.[10] Earl and colleagues[6] reported that tibiotalar joint changes occur after sectioning the superficial deltoid ligament complex. The joint contact area decreased 43%, the peak pressures increased 30%, and the center of rotation moved 4 mm laterally. These findings could contribute to the degeneration and development of osteoarthritis of the tibiotalar joint. This was first stated in a classic biomechanical study by Ramsey and Hamilton,[10] who demonstrated a dramatic decrease in the contact area between the tibia and talus with small displacement with use of a carbon black transference technique, although using some nonphysiologic aspects on their models. This was further explored by Thordarson and coworkers,[11] who evaluated the individual and combined effects of fibular shortening, lateral displacement, and external rotation and found significant increases in the contact pressures in the midlateral and posterolateral quadrants of the talar dome in association with most of the displacement conditions.

Our perspective about the scenario of acute rotational instability is that following an eversion force the talus may forcibly invert in the mortise and as a result injure the medial and lateral ligament complex. This is probably a frequent situation regularly misdiagnosed as an acute lateral sprain without taking into account the medial component, because probably many of the lateral instabilities are in fact rotational.

Worthy of notice is that the term "stability," in the context of a deltoid ligament injury, makes reference to the tibiotalar joint. Although the exact contribution of each fascicle to overall ankle congruity is only proven in cadaver models, far less known is the role of the medial collateral ligament in the subtalar or even Chopart stability.

Could a neglected or not adequately treated injury to the superficial deltoid ligament, or even to its tibionavicular or tibiocalcaneal fascicles, ultimately result in a flat foot? Although this may be just a theoretic concern, we firmly believe that further characterization of the exact role of each individual fascicle is necessary to fully appraise the risk of evolution to chronic hindfoot instability of the acute deltoid lesions.

The contribution of medial ligament disruption to the progressive collapse of the medial arch is discussed in the recent work by Myerson and colleagues,[12] in which not only a novel classification system is proposed but a debate about the different elements that interact in the genesis of the acquired adult flatfoot, historically linked to the posterior tibial tendon lesion.

PATIENT EVALUATION OVERVIEW
Clinical Evaluation

Before examining the patient, it is important to briefly inquire about the injury mechanism. Patients usually tell a history of an eversion trauma, but curiously an inversion trauma followed by external rotation of the talus can also damage the deltoid ligament. The patient also should be specifically asked whether this was a primary trauma or if he or she has sustained earlier ankle sprains, thus the injury may be in the context of a chronic instability. Because this is often not clearly indicated, additional imaging assessment may be considered, such as stress radiographs, MRI, or ultrasound.

Acute injuries of the deltoid complex usually present with medial-sided ankle swelling or hematoma. The anterior portion of the medial malleolus is commonly tender to palpation.[11] However, not only the damaged ligament can be the source of pain: synovitis of the medial part of the ankle joint can be responsible for this symptom too.

Pain and ecchymosis usually reflect ligament injury, but they are not reliable at determining the key issue: medial ankle instability. Unlike lateral ankle instability, these patients do not make reference to "giving way" so frequently, making it difficult to determine if they are unstable or not.

Physical examination for the presence of medial injuries is not reliable in the setting of acute lateral ankle injury.[13] Pain and ecchymosis showed low sensibility and specificity in previous studies.[2]

Lateral ankle instability assessment (stress and drawer tests) and careful syndesmosis evaluation are mandatory, because they are frequently associated.

A thorough examination should include the foot type assessment. It is suggested that flat feet would have a worse prognosis than well aligned feet, because strain onto the medial hind foot soft tissues (eg, deltoid ligament, posterior tibial tendon) could be already present. The bone structure may provide a protective role against progression to a chronic lesion because cavus feet with medial ligament injuries, in the authors' experience, do not develop chronic medial instability.

Images

Standard radiographs are used to exclude fractures after acute trauma. Widening of the medial clear space on a weightbearing mortise view has long been used as a sign of deltoid ligament insufficiency. However, this sign lacks sensitivity in the diagnosis of injuries of the deep layer of the deltoid complex.[14]

A previous arthroscopic study reported a significant false-positive rate of 53.6% for complete tears of the deep deltoid ligament by radiographic widening of the medial clear space (4 mm or more).[14] Cheung and colleagues[15] have reported that medial clear space widening usually correlated with tears of the syndesmotic ligaments and deep deltoid ligament.

Probably the most reliable method in evaluation of deltoid ligament is MRI.[16,17] This imaging method has shown to have a sensitivity of 84% and specificity of 93% when evaluating injury to any portion of the deltoid ligament,[17] and even when considering injuries to the superficial and deep portions separately, specificity and sensitivity remains high.[16]

It is useful to have a systematic routine of examination of the different structures, so as not to miss any injury, especially for the less experienced eye. From anterior to posterior the structures to evaluate are the deltoid ligament, followed by the flexor retinaculum, the spring ligament, and the posterior tibial tendon.[18–21]

A superficial deltoid ligament tear may be seen as a focal discontinuity at its site of origin or as detachment of a sheet of fibrous tissue from the entire superficial aspect of the medial malleolus from anterior to posterior.[16]

The coronal plane assessment allows to evaluate the tibiocalcaneal band of the superficial deltoid, the tibiospring ligament up in the place where it merges with the superomedial band of the spring ligament, and the tibionavicular band located deep to the posterior tibial tendon.[16] In the axial plane analysis, the examiner should recognize the posterior tibiotalar band inserting in the talar body just posterior to the medial malleolus.

This plane also enables the view of the so-called medial malleolar fascial sleeve, a term that defines the merging of the superficial deltoid fibers, the periosteum of the medial malleolus, and the flexor retinaculum (**Fig. 1**).[16,18] The presence of edema, delamination, or complete discontinuity either in its origin or more distally may be seen in an acute injury.

The last element that could be visualized is the tibionavicular band, which is the most anterior portion of the superficial layer; because this runs in an oblique fashion it cannot be fully depicted in coronal or axial images. In this case three-dimensional sequences are useful.[16] In fluid-sensitive images it is normal to see a small amount of high signal intensity between the fibers, which gives the ligament a striated appearance, although the individual fibers should always appear taut and sharply

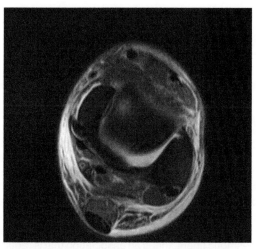

Fig. 1. MRI axial view showing the medial facial sleeve detachment.

demarcated.[16] When injured, the ligament may displace slightly superiorly (**Fig. 2**). Osseous edema in the talar footprint of the deep deltoid ligament insertion may also be seen. This image should not be confused with medial joint line bone bruising, which may be seen together with lateral ligamentous injuries usually caused by contrecoup impaction[16] and rotational forces during an inversion injury,[22] which is significantly associated with an anterior inferior tibiofibular ligament tear.[23]

Despite MRI sensitivity its static nature makes it unable to assess joint stability.[24] Ultrasonography could discriminate the injured layer and the site of the lesion, while allowing to perform dynamic maneuvers.[25] It also yields a rapid comparison with the asymptomatic ankle. In a study by Rosa and colleagues,[24] ultrasonography was a highly accurate diagnostic modality (100% sensitivity, 90% specificity, 97% positive

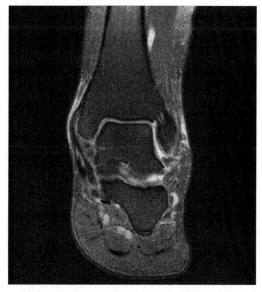

Fig. 2. MRI depicting the loose of striated appearance of deep tibiotalar ligament.

predictive value, and 100% negative predictive value) in the assessment of deltoid ligaments in the setting of an ankle fracture.

Injuries of the superficial layer of the medial collateral ligament complex have been classified in the orthopedic literature by the level of lesion[2]: type I injuries, in which there is a proximal tear or avulsion of the deltoid ligament, are by far the most frequent (71%); type II injuries, in which there is a midsubstance tear (10%), and type III injuries, in which there is a distal tear (19%), are both less frequent.

Associated Lesions

An associated lesion of the flexor retinaculum could be found because of the proximity of its periosteal attachment to the origin of the superficial layer of the medial collateral ligament complex.[26] Thickening greater than 2 mm, periosteal detachment, and even interruption can be seen. Because of the high incidence of associated lesions, the spring ligament complex, the syndesmosis, and the lateral ligaments should all be carefully evaluated.

Because the mechanism of injury needed to damage the deltoid ligament fibers could also impair the syndesmotic fibers, this is an association that is required to be ruled out. Diagnosing syndesmotic instability is challenging because of the three-dimensional nature of distal fibular motion after injury, which may be coronal, sagittal, or rotational.[27]

The most common associated injury is the lateral collateral ligament tear.[27,28]

ELEMENTS FOR DECISION MAKING

The optimal way of treat these group of patients has yet to be defined. There is a lack of evidence about how to manage isolated medial ankle lesions. To begin with, it is mandatory to rule out any associated fracture and/or associated ligamentous injury.

Once the ligament injury is identified, the most important aspect is to determine whether the lesion alters or not the tibiotalar stability, by analyzing weightbearing radiographs. We define a stable lesion as one that does not alter the medial clear space in anteroposterior and mortise weightbearing comparative views. Additionally, one must check if the patient had previous medial or lateral instability. The second issue is to take into consideration the patient's characteristics (eg, age, activity level).

We also may address the foot type to consider its influence in the prognosis. For this purpose, we routinely use weightbearing radiographs and MRI images to recognize foot deformity and to characterize the type of ligament injury and the compromised fascicles, which may indicate instability. It is also mandatory to rule out syndesmosis lesions, lateral ligament damage, and the presence of associated chondral lesions.

Stable lesions are best treated conservatively, yet the optimal treatment of unstable lesions is controversial. Most of the evidence is supported by ankle fracture studies, which sustain that surgery does not yield better results than conservative treatment.[29] The authors' preference is to treat young and active patients with an arthroscopy (to rule out additional pathologies) and open ligament repair, and elder and less active patients with conservative treatment (**Fig. 3**).

AUTHORS' PREFERRED METHOD OF TREATMENT
Nonsurgical Treatment

Conservative treatment is the mainstay of treatment of stable lesions. It is also a good option for unstable cases, particularly in less active patients. Curiously, in most of the studies, "conservative" means "nonsurgical," missing out on a thorough description of a proper conservative treatment.

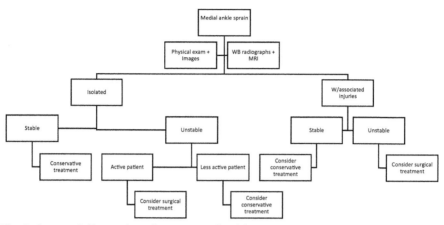

Fig. 3. Proposed diagnostic and treatment algorithm.

Immobilization

The immobilization type is not enough appraised in the literature. The posterior tibio-talar ligament is tight when the foot is in 90°, such as when weightbearing on a plan-tigrade foot, and loose when the foot is plantar flexed.[30] Although a walker boot is commonly used (stable injuries), a cast is the best option for unstable or borderline in-juries to obtain an adequate ligament healing with the proper length. Walker boots are often taken in and out by patients, allowing an overlengthened deltoid ligament, which leads to chronic instability.

A 6-week period of immobilization is necessary (the last 2 weeks with a removable boot to allow physical therapy). Return to previous sporting activities is progressively allowed at 16 weeks and may be accompanied by medial discomfort in some patients.

Weightbearing

Weightbearing is a controversial topic that lacks current evidence. Difficulties arise in how to assess which fascicles are torn and consequently if the lesion is stable or not. It is helpful to obtain weightbearing radiographs to assess stability. If the medial clear space is normal, one can assume we are facing a stable lesion and weightbearing is allowed. Conversely, if medial clear space widening is observed, surgical treatment is indicated.

Once the ligament is healed, if the patient has a flat foot or even a moderate hyper-pronation it is helpful to prescribe a foot orthosis with a medial longitudinal arch (with medial post in flat foot cases). They usually alleviate the medial hindfoot soft tissue strain (eg, deltoid ligament, posterior tibial tendon), that normally bothers the patient for many weeks.

Physical therapy should be initiated at 3 weeks if a walker boot is used, and at 4 weeks if a cast was indicated. Ankle dorsiflexion should be encouraged to prevent anteromedial ankle impingement, which is a common complication in these cases. A proprioception training is also necessary to improve stability.

SURGICAL TREATMENT

Although most medial ankle sprains are mild to moderate and can be treated nonop-eratively, an increasing number of patients are being recognized with more severe in-juries leading to prolonged medial ankle instability.[31] In these patients, surgical repair or reconstruction of the deltoid ligament may be required to restore medial ankle stability.[31]

We routinely begin with an arthroscopy to properly identify the deltoid ligament damage (**Figs. 4**A, B and **5**), and to diagnose and treat any other lesion.

Injuries to the deltoid ligament usually occur at the proximal insertion site, and its insertion zone at the medial malleolus shows a naked area of periosteum where the ligament is detached. Furthermore, associated cartilage lesions can be identified. We then proceed to reattach the injured deltoid ligament.

Surgical Technique

Although previous reports on arthroscopic repair[7] have been published by surgeons with extensive experience, we believe that arthroscopic techniques limit the repair to the superficial fascicles. Therefore, we proceed with the open repair technique after the arthroscopy.

On the medial side, a gently curved incision 4 to 8 cm long is made, starting 1 to 2 cm cranially of the tip of the medial malleolus toward the medial aspect of the navicular. After dissection of the fascia, the anterior aspect of the deltoid ligament is exposed. The tibionavicular ligament and the tibiospring ligament can also be explored.

A complete acute rupture often occurs in the proximal portion of the deltoid ligament. Reinsertion to the medial malleolus is achieved by suturing directly to the bone. According to the site and extent of the rupture, one or two suture anchors were placed in the medial malleolus, 5 mm lateral to the cartilage or medial aspect of talus. Suture anchors were buried slightly below the bony surface, and FiberWire sutures were used to create a full-thickness, horizontal mattress suture pattern in the deltoid ligament complex for a direct repair (**Fig. 6**). During the repair, the ankle was slightly inverted to reduce tension on the deltoid complex repair. Once the sutures

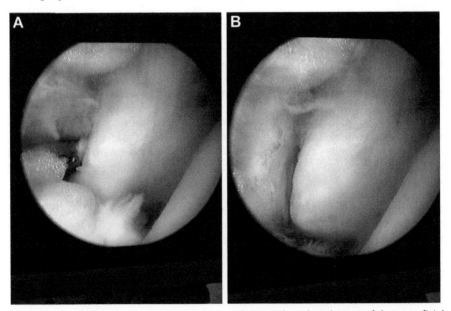

Fig. 4. (A, B) Arthroscopic image demonstrating the complete detachment of the superficial tibionavicular ligament with and without introducing a Halsted in the created space.

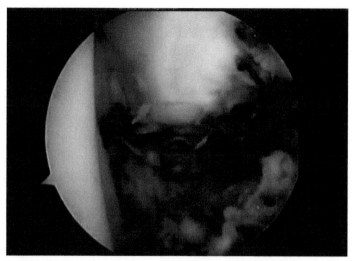

Fig. 5. Arthroscopic image of a completely torn deep deltoid ligament.

from the anchor had been placed and the appropriate tension was applied, the surrounding soft tissues were imbricated to provide additional support.

Postoperative Protocol

All patients followed a standardized rehabilitation protocol consisting of being non-weightbearing in a cast for 2 to 4 weeks. From 4 to 6 weeks, patients were transitioned into a boot brace with progression of weightbearing. Physical therapy was started 4 weeks postoperatively, with range of motion and stretching. Ankle dorsiflexion should be encouraged to prevent anteromedial ankle impingement, which is a common complication in these cases. Proprioception training is also necessary to improve stability.

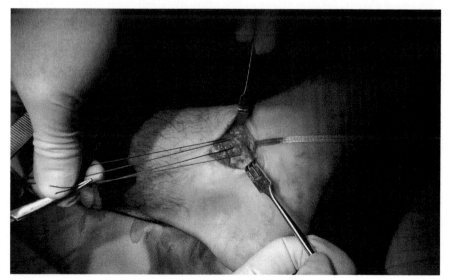

Fig. 6. Direct repair of the detached deltoid ligament.

COMPLICATIONS

- Chronic medial ankle instability: Neglected injuries or inadequate treatments frequently leads to chronic instability. It is important to remark that this situation is much more probable to occur than in lateral ankle sprains. With that stated, a proper diagnosis cannot be overemphasized.
- Anteromedial impingement: This is also a frequent scenario, particularly in conservative treatment, when patients undergo a prolonged period of immobilization. Early range of motion is the best recommendation to avoid it. In symptomatic cases, an arthroscopic debridement is indicated to remove the scar tissue in the superomedial corner of the ankle joint.
- Acquired flat foot deformity: This deformity can occur in neglected cases. After a failed conservative treatment trial (eg, orthosis), reconstructive surgery may be indicated (including osteotomies to restore bony alignment).
- Medial ankle pain: Patients commonly complain about medial ankle pain for several weeks or months. Frequently a posterior tibial tenosynovitis is the main cause. If symptoms persist, the hindfoot alignment may be addressed to unload the stress to the posterior tibial as the main invertor of the hindfoot. Not uncommonly, the situation is more complex, and sometimes it is necessary to undergo a flat foot reconstruction to alleviate symptoms.

NEW DEVELOPMENTS

A novel idea to reduce immobilization time, is to enhance the surgical repair with a device that protects and augments the sutures (**Fig. 7**), placed extra-articular once the ligament is repaired, and may allow to encourage the patient to perform early range of motion.[32] Consequently, this might reduce the chance of scar tissue developing, the main etiologic factor of anterior ankle impingement. However, publications in this sense are still case series of patients with chronic medial instability.

TREATMENT EVIDENCE

Evidence confronting surgical versus conservative treatment in acute deltoid ligament lesions is largely anchored in the setting of ankle fractures; extrapolation of results

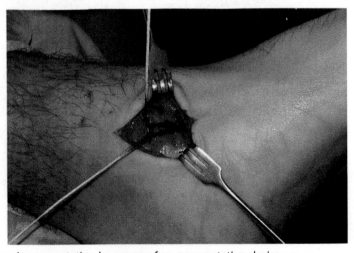

Fig. 7. Repair augmentation by means of an augmentation device.

may be done when analyzing the treatment possibilities in isolated deltoid lesions. Previous results showed no differences in subjective or objective outcomes with deltoid repair during ankle fracture fixation compared with nonoperative deltoid management.[33,34] There are currently few objective data in the literature regarding medial ankle instability after either conservative or surgical treatment of acute deltoid injuries. Ultimately treatment decision relies on the clinical and image appraisal of each individual patient.

CLINICS CARE POINTS

- Deltoid ligament injuries in a valgus ankle could potentially lead to a chronic medial instability because of the previous tissue strain.

- When evaluating a medial ankle sprain and finding valgus talar tilt, look for associated syndesmotic or lateral ligament injury.

- Choosing for nonsurgical treatment involves a 6-week period of strict immobilization; consider nonweightbearing the first 4 weeks, followed by a physical therapy program.

- Following either election of treatment in patients with overpronation or valgus hindfoot consider a foot orthosis with medial arch support.

DISCLOSURE

The authors have nothing to disclose.

REFERENCES

1. Waterman BR, Belmont PJ Jr, Cameron KL, et al. Risk factors for syndesmotic and medial ankle sprain: role of sex, sport, and level of competition. Am J Sports Med 2011;39(5):992–8.
2. Hintermann B, Knupp M, Pagenstert GI. Deltoid ligament injuries: diagnosis and management. Foot Ankle Clin 2006;11:625–37.
3. Lotscher P, Lang TH, Zwicky L, et al. Osteoligamentous injuries of the medial ankle joint. Eur J Trauma Emerg Surg 2015;41:615–21.
4. Ferran NA, Maffulli N. Epidemiology of sprains of the lateral ankle ligament complex. Foot Ankle Clin N Am 2006;11:659–62.
5. Bi C, Kong D, Lin J, et al. Diagnostic value of intraoperative tap test for acute deltoid ligament injury. Eur J Trauma Emerg Surg 2019. https://doi.org/10.1007/s00068-019-01243-w.
6. Earl M, Wayne J, Brodrick C, et al. Contribution of the deltoid ligament to ankle joint contact characteristics: a cadaver study. Foot Ankle Int 1996;17:317–24.
7. Acevedo JI, Kreulen C, Cedeno AA, et al. Technique for arthroscopic deltoid ligament repair with description of safe zones. Foot Ankle Int 2020. https://doi.org/10.1177/1071100720909138. 107110072090913.
8. Clanton TO, Williams BT, James EW, et al. Radiographic identification of the deltoid ligament complex of the medial ankle. Am J Sports Med 2015;43(11):2753–62.
9. Jackson R, Wills RE, Jackson R. Rupture of deltoid ligament without involvement of the lateral ligament. Am J Sports Med 1988;16:541–3.
10. Ramsey PL, Hamilton W. Changes in tibiotalar area of contact caused by lateral talar shift. J Bone Joint Surg Am 1976;58(3):356–7.

11. Thordarson DB, Motamed S, Hedman T, et al. The effect of fibular malreduction on contact pressures in an ankle fracture malunion model. J Bone Joint Surg Am 1997;79(12):1809–15.

12. Myerson MS, Thordarson DB, Johnson JE, et al. Classification and nomenclature: progressive collapsing foot deformity. Foot Ankle Int 2020;41(10):1271–6.

13. Chhabra A, Subhawong TK, Carrino JA. MR imaging of deltoid ligament pathologic findings and associated impingement syndromes. Radiographics 2010; 30(3):751–61.

14. van den Bekerom MP, Mutsaerts EL, van Dijk CN. Evaluation of the integrity of the deltoid ligament in supination external rotation ankle fractures: a systematic review of the literature. Arch Orthop Trauma Surg 2009;129:227–35.

15. Cheung Y, Perrich KD, Gui J, et al. MRI of isolated distal fibular fractures with widened medial clear space on stressed radiographs: which ligaments are interrupted? AJR Am J Roentgenol 2009;192(1):W7–12.

16. Schuberth JM, Collman DR, Rush SM, et al. Deltoid ligament integrity in lateral malleolar fractures: a comparative analysis of arthroscopic and radiographic assessments. J Foot Ankle Surg 2004;43(1):20–9.

17. Crim J, Longenecker LG. MRI and surgical findings in deltoid ligament tears. AJR Am J Roentgenol 2015;204:W63–9.

18. Chun KY, Choi YS, Lee SH, et al. Deltoid ligament and tibiofibular syndesmosis injury in chronic lateral ankle instability: magnetic resonance imaging evaluation at 3T and comparison with arthroscopy. Korean J Radiol 2015;16:1096–103.

19. Crim J. Medial-sided ankle pain: deltoid ligament and beyond. Magn Reson Imaging Clin N Am 2017;25(1):63–77.

20. Duc SR, Mengiardi B, Pfirrmann CWA, et al. Improved visualization of collateral ligaments of the ankle: multiplanar reconstructions based on standard 2D turbo spin-echo MR images. Eur Radiol 2007;17(5):1162–71.

21. Klein MA. MR imaging of the ankle: normal and abnormal findings in the medial collateral ligament. AJR Am J Roentgenol 1994;162(2):377–83.

22. Mengiardi B, Pinto C, Zanetti M. Medial collateral ligament complex of the ankle: MR imaging anatomy and findings in medial instability. Semin Musculoskelet Radiol 2016;20(1):91–103.

23. Sanders TG, Medynski MA, Feller JF, et al. Bone contusion patterns of the knee at MR imaging: footprint of the mechanism of injury. Radiographics 2000;20: S135e51.

24. Rosa I, Rodeia J, Fernandes PX, et al. Ultrasonographic assessment of deltoid ligament integrity in ankle fractures. Foot Ankle Int 2020;41(2):147–53.

25. Park JW, Lee SJ, Choo HJ, et al. Ultrasonography of the ankle joint. Ultrasonography 2017;36:321–35.

26. Sconfienza LM, Orlandi D, Lacelli F, et al. Dynamic high-resolution US of ankle and midfoot ligaments: normal anatomic structure and imaging technique. Radiographics 2015;35(1):164–78.

27. Numkarunarunrote N, Malik A, Aguiar RO, et al. Retinacula of the foot and ankle: MRI with anatomic correlation in cadavers. AJR Am J Roentgenol 2007;188(4): W348–54.

28. Crim JR, Beals TC, Nickisch F, et al. Deltoid ligament abnormalities in chronic lateral ankle instability. Foot Ankle Int 2011;32:873–8.

29. Hintermann B, Regazzoni P, Lampert C, et al. Arthroscopic findings in acute fractures of the ankle. J Bone Joint Surg Br 2000;82:345–51.

30. Savage-Elliott I, Murawski CD, Smyth NA, et al. The deltoid ligament: an in-depth review of anatomy, function, and treatment strategies. Knee Surg Sports Traumatol Arthrosc 2013;21:1316–27.
31. Gougoulias N, Sakellariou A. When is a simple fracture of the lateral malleolus not so simple? how to assess stability, which ones to fix and the role of the deltoid ligament. Bone Joint J 2017;99-B(7):851–5.
32. Hintermann B, Valderrabano V, Boss A, et al. Medial ankle instability: an exploratory, prospective study of fifty-two cases. Am J Sports Med 2004;32:183–90.
33. Pellegrini MJ, Torres N, Cuchacovich NR, et al. Chronic deltoid ligament insufficiency repair with Internal Brace™ augmentation. Foot Ankle Surg 2019;25(6): 812–8.
34. Berkes MB, Little MT, Lazaro LE, et al. Malleolar fractures and their ligamentous injury equivalents have similar outcomes in supination-external rotation type IV fractures of the ankle treated by anatomical internal fixation. J Bone Joint Surg Br 2012;94(11):1567–72.

State of the Art in Treatment of Chronic Medial Ankle Instability

Cesar de Cesar Netto, MD, PhD*, John E. Femino, MD

KEYWORDS

- Deltoid ligament • Deltoid instability • Ankle instability • Chronic deltoid instability
- Chronic medial ankle instability • Multidirectional ankle instability

KEY POINTS

- The deltoid ligament complex represents a primary and crucial stabilizer of the ankle joint and comprises 2 layers and 6 main components.
- The key mechanism for deltoid ligament injury is eversion and/or external rotation trauma of the ankle, and association with syndesmotic injury is frequent.
- Chronic deltoid instability can potentially lead to posttraumatic osteoarthritis of the ankle.
- Proper diagnosis and treatment of chronic deltoid instability is crucial for long-term outcomes.
- Surgical treatment of chronic deltoid instability is frequently needed, and multiple surgical techniques have been described.

INTRODUCTION

Posttraumatic osteoarthritis of the ankle (PTOA) is a disabling condition that has been shown to have negative impact on quality of life comparable with other major chronic medical conditions such as end-stage kidney disease and chronic heart failure.[1] PTOA also has similar physical and mental disability measures to osteoarthritis of the hip.[2] Regarding PTOA epidemiology, Saltzman and colleagues[3] reported on 445 patients with PTOA and revealed that the 3 most common traumatic causes were related to history of prior rotational ankle fractures (37%), ligamentous ankle instability (28.3%, 14.6% secondary to recurrent instability and 13.7% resulting from a single ankle sprain), and tibial plafond fractures (9%). The investigators did not mention chronic deltoid instability (CDI) as causative factor for PTOA.

Foot and Ankle Services, Department of Orthopedics and Rehabilitation, University of Iowa, Carver College of Medicine, John Pappajohn Pavilion (JPP), Room 01066, Lower Level, 200 Hawkins Drive, Iowa City, IA 52242, USA
* Corresponding author.
E-mail address: Cesar-netto@uiowa.edu
Twitter: @Dr_deCesarNetto (C.C.N.)

Foot Ankle Clin N Am 26 (2021) 329–344
https://doi.org/10.1016/j.fcl.2021.03.007
1083-7515/21/© 2021 Elsevier Inc. All rights reserved.

foot.theclinics.com

The specific role of deltoid ligament injury and CDI leading to PTOA is frequently overlooked and underreported in the literature,[4–6] despite the paramount function of the superficial and deep components of the ligament in the overall stability of the ankle joint. In 1956, Close[7] pointed out in a classic and landmark cadaveric and biomechanical study that the sectioning of the deep deltoid ligament (DDL) fibers was decisive in producing marked ankle and syndesmotic instability,[7] where no more than 2 mm of separation between the talus and medial malleolus would occur when the DDL fibers were intact. Twenty years later, Ramsey and Hamilton,[9] in another groundbreaking study, showed that, with a minimal lateral translation of the talus underneath the ankle mortise of 1 mm, the contact area of the ankle joint markedly decreased by 42%, potentially importantly altering the mechanics of the joint. More recently, Burns and colleagues[8] corroborated with the results of the 2 prior studies, showing that only after sectioning of the deltoid ligament does a significant reduction in tibiotalar contact area (39%) and increase in ankle peak pressures (42%) occur. Combined interpretation of the results of these studies highlights the anatomic and biomechanical properties of the deltoid ligament in the stability of the ankle joint and the potential significance of CDI in the development of PTOA.[7–9]

This article not only summarizes the most important anatomic and biomechanical properties of the deltoid ligament complex but highlights the potential role of CDI in the development of PTOA, and the unequivocal importance of optimal diagnosis and treatment of patients with CDI.

Anatomy and Function of the Deltoid Ligament Complex

The deltoid ligament complex is a delta-shaped, strong, broad, and multifascicular ligament that spans out of the medial malleolus to the talus, calcaneus, and navicular bones. It is a primary medial stabilizer of the ankle joint and restricts valgus tilt and anterior and lateral translation of the talus. It has been described in varied ways but it is composed of 2 layers with 6 main components.[10–12] The superficial deltoid ligament (SDL) layer has a total of 4 components that frequently blend into each other. Its main function is to resist eversion of the hindfoot.[13] The tibionavicular component expands anteriorly and connects the anterior medial malleolus to the navicular. It prevents anterior subluxation of the medial talus and it functions as a major support of the spring ligament complex. The fibers become progressively more tensioned with plantarflexion of the ankle joint, starting at 10°.[12] The tibiospring component also arises from the anterior aspect of the medial malleolus and blends distally with the spring ligament complex. Its fibers also become gradually more tensioned with plantar flexion, starting at 15°.[12] The tibiocalcaneal component ($_{TC}$SDL) is the strongest of the superficial ligaments, arising from the medial aspect of the anterior colliculus of the medial malleolus and inserting onto the medial sustentaculum tali. It functions essentially as a true collateral ligament of the ankle, analogous to the medial collateral ligament of the knee (**Fig. 1**). The $_{TC}$SDL fibers are tensioned with ankle dorsiflexion starting at 0°.[12] The posterior component of the SDL arises from the medial aspect of the medial malleolus posterior colliculus and has a broad insertion to the posterior aspect of the talus, blending with fibers of the posterior component of the DDL (pDDL). Its fibers also become progressively more tensioned after 0° of dorsiflexion.[12]

The DDL is the primary restrainer to external rotation of the talus.[13] However, it has 2 different components with particular distinctive functions. The anterior DDL (aDDL) arises from the inferior surface of the medial malleolar anterior colliculus and intercollicular fossa, inserting anteriorly in a corresponding fossa on the medial talus adjacent to the talar body-neck junction. It resists external rotation of the talus (or internal rotation of the tibia on a fixed talus in stance phase of gait) (see **Fig. 1**). It functions in

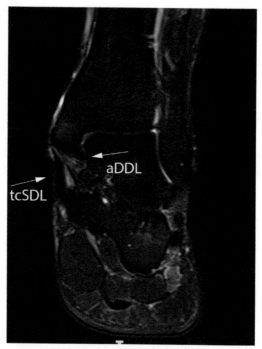

Fig. 1. Coronal plane MRI fat-saturated image depicting the anterior deep deltoid ligament (aDDL) and the tcSDL. Note that aDDL has a broad insertion in the fossa below the articular surface of the medial gutter. The fiber orientation in the coronal plane is optimized to resist external rotation of the talus or internal rotation of the tibia on a fixed talus as during stance phase of gait. The aDDL is coupled with the syndesmosis in resisting talar external rotation. The tcSDL spans the ankle in a vertical orientation and functions like a collateral ligament resisting valgus as the medial collateral ligament would at the knee.

conjunction with the anterior tibiofibular ligament in resisting external rotation forces of the talus and fibula. The pDDL spans from the intercollicular fossa and deep portion of the posterior colliculus into the medial aspect of the talar body in the posterior portion of the medial talar fossa; it resists posterior translation of the talus from under the tibia or anterior translation of the tibia on a fixed talus. In plantarflexion, it is vertical relative to the tibial axis and the fibers are relaxed. In ankle dorsiflexion, the fibers assume an oblique sagittal orientation and become tense as the talus rolls back into the mortise with dorsiflexion (**Fig. 2**).

Mechanism and Long-term Outcomes of Injuries of the Deltoid Ligament Complex

The medial and lateral collateral ligament complexes of the ankle joint provide around 70% of rotational stability in the transverse plane,[14] particularly when the ankle is in a plantarflexed position, whereas the sagittal and coronal plane stability are mainly supported by the extremely congruent anatomy of the ankle joint, more importantly in a neutrally dorsiflexed position.[15]

The key mechanism of deltoid ligament injury in the acute setting is eversion and/or external rotation of the ankle, or more precisely eversion and internal rotation of the leg in a plantigrade and weight-bearing fixed foot.[16] The injury pattern can happen in multiple traumatic scenarios, including isolated medial ankle sprains (reported incidence

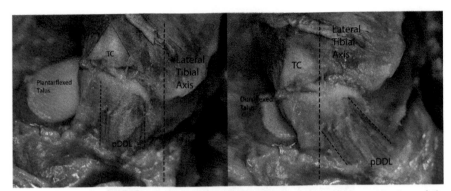

Fig. 2. Cadaveric anatomic dissection of the medial ankle showing the positioning of the pDDL fibers, which become tense with dorsiflexion of the ankle. The tcSDL (TC) was resected. The orientation of the ligament changes from a relaxed vertical orientation (*left*) to a tense sagittal orientation when the ankle is dorsiflexed (*right*). The functional stabilization of the tibia on the fixed talus prevents anterior translation of the tibia from heel strike through heel-off.

of 5%–15% of all ankle sprains),[17,18] concomitantly to lateral ankle sprains[6,19] and in association with rotational ankle fractures.[20] Additional injuries occurring alongside deltoid injuries include fibular fractures, syndesmotic injuries, and osteochondral injuries of the talar dome and distal tibia.[11]

In a biomechanical study, transection of the SDL was compared with transection of the DDL each in combination with a fibular osteotomy.[21] Significant external rotation with associated medial clear space widening only occurred following DDL transection. Another biomechanical study using three-dimensional computed tomography analysis evaluated the effect of hindfoot position on external rotation stress.[22] Either varus or valgus hindfoot position (varus being more effective) was able to produce statistically significant external rotation of the talus in the condition of a transected DDL alone. This finding suggests that abnormal kinematics of the talus within an intact mortise would exist even when a fibula fracture with or without a syndesmosis injury was anatomically reduced. This scenario is realistic considering that the DDL is rarely visualized with most operatively treated ankle fractures without a medial malleolus fracture. It is an intra-articular ligament like the anterior cruciate ligament (ACL) of the knee and emphasizes the importance of the DDL in the overall ankle instability. It has also been shown that synovial cells can affect gene expression of myofibroblasts to cause retraction of the torn ACL stumps leading to failure of healing.[23] It is hard to imagine the intra-articular DDL healing any better following a traumatic injury.

With these concepts in mind, it is also important to acknowledge the frequently combined injury of deltoid and syndesmotic ligament complexes. Malreductions of the tibiofibular syndesmosis in operatively treated ankle fractures have been shown to lead to worse clinical and radiographic outcomes.[24,25] Medial clear space radiographic widening is usually used as a proxy for not just deltoid ligament but also for syndesmotic injury.[26–28] In an analysis of reoperations because of malreduction of ankle fractures, the most common indication for reoperation was malreduction of the syndesmosis (59%).[29] Contrasting with syndesmotic injuries/instability, long-term findings and outcomes of patients with residual deltoid ligament instability are unknown.[30]

A systematic review of 1822 operatively treated ankle fractures revealed that only 79.3% of patients who were deemed to have optimally reduced fractures had good to excellent outcomes; the remainder experienced joint degeneration with unknown causes.[31] This finding of 20% poor outcomes in otherwise radiographically satisfactory ankle fracture reductions is remarkable. The weakness of the literature in this area is highlighted by grade B and C value conclusions. Most cases of symptomatic ankle osteoarthritis are found in patients who have previously experienced low-energy rotational ankle fractures or recurrent ankle sprains.[3,32] Among patients with PTOA, the latency time between injury and presentation to a specialty clinic with end-stage PTOA was 20.9 years (1–52 years).[33] It is reasonable to suppose that one of the potential causes of progression of joint degeneration is related to residual rotational instability and deltoid ligament instability, mainly of the DDL.

Patient Evaluation and Management Overview

CDI symptoms can be difficult for patients to describe and localize because they are usually more subtle than lateral ankle ligament instability.[34] Symptoms of lateral ankle pain associated with syndesmotic instability may be combined with medial ankle symptoms.[19] Physical examination tests such as the leg compression test, fibula drawer, and external rotation stress test can be helpful in confirming syndesmotic instability.[35] Tenderness over the medial gutter and at the medial inframalleolar area are moderate indicators of deltoid ligament complex injury.[36] Three classic maneuvers are described for deltoid ligament injury and residual medial instability: valgus stress, anteromedial drawer, and Kleiger tests.[37] Detection of medial ankle instability may be aided by a varus external rotation stress test, which can elicit medial pain as well as lateral pain caused by an unstable syndesmosis.[38] Analogous to the lateral ankle, an anterior drawer test of the medial ankle with hindfoot varus can also detect deep deltoid instability with pain or apprehension.[22] In a normal ankle, there should be little to no anterior translation with drawer stress; however, in the unstable ankle, the translation can approach 10 mm. Although the authors have found these to be helpful in our practice, it is important to acknowledge that these tests have not been validated clinically. However, the varus external rotation stress test does have a strong basis in biomechanical analysis.[22,38] The use of weight-bearing computed tomography (WBCT) has also recently been shown to represent an important diagnostic tool for subtle syndesmotic instability and can potentially represent an interesting option for diagnosing mild CDI.[39–44] MRI, particularly in the coronal plane, can show the anatomy of the deltoid ligament complex clearly, and can serve as an adjunctive diagnostic tool for deltoid ligament injury and potential residual instability.[45]

Patients with chronic residual deltoid instability should always be treated with a good trial of nonoperative measures, including bracing and orthotics for stability or alignment problems, as well as physical therapy for inversion and eversion strengthening.[11,46] Nonsteroidal antiinflammatory medications can also be helpful in some cases. Operative treatment is considered when patients fail to achieve satisfactory pain relief with nonoperative measures or in cases with significant instability.[4,11,47]

Surgical treatment of patients for CDI should always be contemplated whenever reconstruction of a chronic syndesmosis injury is being considered.[4] Patients with advanced PTOA are best treated with ankle arthrodesis or total ankle arthroplasty. In patients with moderate degenerative changes and impingement, with minimal mid-range motion pain, ligament reconstruction can be performed with joint-sparing osteotomies and arthroscopic debridement for impingement. The timeline to future ankle replacement should always be a consideration because drill holes and tunnels in the talus can compromise vascularity.[48] Multiple techniques for superficial and DDL repair/reconstruction have been described in the literature, most of them focusing on either the acute setting[30,46,49–55] or reconstruction techniques for cases of progressive collapsing foot deformity[56,57] (also called adult acquired flatfoot deformity) with valgus tilting of the ankle joint.[58–66]

Only a few articles describe specific surgical techniques in the setting of multidirectional ankle instability or isolated CDI.[4,67,68]

Operative Procedure (Authors' Favorite Technique)

The technique for deltoid ligament reconstruction described here is similar to one previously reported for acute deltoid injuries and concomitant syndesmotic disruption,[69] with the exception being that the FiberTape is combined with a thin autograft or allograft tendon (3–4 mm) to provide soft tissue augmentation for the chronically disrupted DDL fibers.

The procedure begins with a diagnostic anterior ankle arthroscopy to confirm the findings of ligamentous instability and to treat associated soft tissue or bony impingement and to evaluate for other intra-articular problems such as osteochondral or purely chondral lesions not previously detected. Examination of the medial gutter space and syndesmotic space under manual external rotation stress, while keeping the hindfoot in varus and the ankle joint in neutral dorsiflexion, is performed (**Fig. 3**).[22,38] Attempts to insert a 2.5-mm and a 3.0-mm arthroscopic sphere in the syndesmotic incisura are performed, with and without the external rotation stress. A positive test for syndesmotic instability is considered when the 3-mm arthroscopic sphere

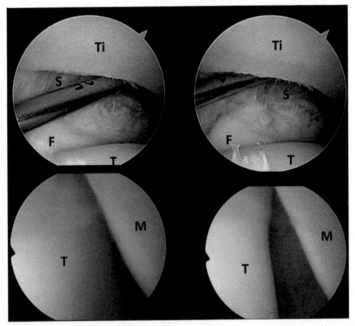

Fig. 3. Arthroscopic assessment of the syndesmotic (*top*) and medial gutter (*bottom*) spaces. Syndesmotic instability is tested under manual external rotation stress of the ankle while keeping the hindfoot in varus. First, a 2.5-mm diameter arthroscopic sphere (*top left*) and then a 3.0-mm diameter arthroscopic sphere (*top right*) are inserted into the syndesmotic space. If the 3.0-mm diameter sphere can be introduced into the incisura, an option is made for open reduction and internal fixation of the syndesmosis. Medial gutter space assessed arthroscopically without (*bottom left*) and with external rotation stress (*bottom right*), showing major instability of the anterior deep deltoid component. F, Fibula; M, Medial Malleolus; S, Syndesmotic Joint; T, Talus; Ti, Tibia.

can be inserted in the syndesmotic space,[70] and in that scenario an open reduction and internal fixation of the syndesmosis with 2 divergent suture button devices is usually performed. Screw fixation is considered for morbidly obese patients or significantly unstable injuries. Anterior drawer and varus stress tests under fluoroscopic guidance is also performed to diagnose concomitant lateral ankle instability.[37]

If syndesmotic fixation is needed, surgical exposure and preparation can be performed at this point, but no reduction/fixation is advisable before preparation of the medial side. The medial ankle can then be opened along a longitudinal incision over the posterior one-third of the medial malleolus and at the level of the intercollicular fossa. Incision is then directed toward the navicular along the dorsal margin of the posterior tibialis tendon sheath. The SDL can be sharply elevated from the medial malleolus proximal to the insertion of the tcSDL on the malleolus, with a transverse incision that is carried to the anterior surface of the medial malleolus (**Fig. 4**). The retinacular/periosteal layer of the local soft tissues is typically thicker than normal because of the fibrosis of healing. This technique usually provides a sufficiently robust flap for later repair augmentation. The SDL is then progressively elevated toward the insertion on the navicular. The retinacular/periosteal/ligamentous sleeve is reflected inferiorly and can later be directly repaired to the convex surface of the malleolus, with small suture anchors as necessary. The insertion of the DDL on the talus is a fossa that is inferior to the comma-shaped articular cartilage of the medial facet of the talar dome, which can be debrided of fibrotic tissue and synovium that can be present in the absence of normal DDL fibers, and sometimes marginal osteophytes may also require removal. In cases where the pDDL requires reconstruction, a guidewire is placed into the posterior portion of the fossa and can be checked on fluoroscopy for direction relative to the articular surfaces of the ankle and subtalar joint (**Fig. 5**).

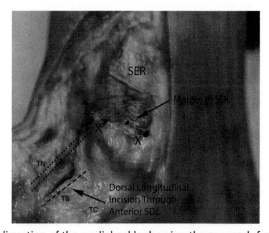

Fig. 4. Anatomic dissection of the medial ankle showing the approach for anatomic deltoid reconstruction by developing a flap of the SDL. The tibial origin of the anterior aspect of the SDL (tibionavicular [TN], tibiospring [TS], and tibiocalcaneal [TC]) is subperiosteally elevated from the medial malleolus. Distally the SDL is incised longitudinally for later primary repair (usually in between TN and TS fibers). The thick periosteal/retinacular layer superior to this provides for primary repair and advancement, which can be augmented by small suture anchors (X). In this case, these tissues were resected to better show the flap (superior extensor retinaculum [SER], cut). In the case of a combined flatfoot reconstruction, the addition of a spring ligament reconstruction can be augmented by an anchor–suture tape construct from the medial malleolus to the navicular (*dotted lines*).

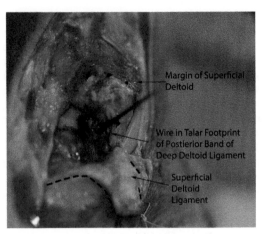

Fig. 5. Anatomic dissection of the anterior medial ankle with the SDL reflected inferiorly showing the positioning of the tunnel for reconstruction of the posterior DDL fibers. Tunnel can be made with a cannulated drill or reamer to ensure precise placement in the hard bone of the posterior talus, distal to the margin of the medial articular talar surface. In this case, the specimen had a small avulsion fracture of the anterior colliculus (A) and deep deltoid insufficiency.

Typically, a 3.9-mm polyether ether ketone (PEEK) anchor is used for the posterior anchor. A 4.5-mm to 5.0-mm reamer for a biotenodesis screw is then used over the guidewire to create a tunnel; the tunnel diameter depends on bone density and graft size. The tunnel is reamed to a depth of 20 mm to accommodate the depth of the anchor plus the graft. A tap can be used to facilitate introduction of the tendon and hardware. Our preference is to use a hamstring allograft or a local extensor digitorum longus tendon (EDL) autograft, harvested at the level of the inferior extensor retinaculum, proximal to its quadrification. The graft/FiberTape construct is then prepared in the back table, with a 0-FiberWire, tubularizing the tendon graft, which is then sewn to the FiberTape, keeping both under manual tension. An ACL graft preparation vice can also be used to maintain graft tension while the FiberTape is sutured to it. The FiberTape is biased to allow for placement of 2 contiguous limbs. The FiberTape and FiberWire sutures are then passed through the eyelet of the anchor (**Fig. 6**) and the posterior limb of the tape-graft construct is implanted with tension on both the Fiber-Tape and FiberWire. The second tunnel is reamed in the intercollicular medial malleolar fossa, just posterior to the tip of the anterior colliculus. The guidewire maintains the exact location of the tunnel. Thumb syndesmotic reduction under direct visualization and fixation can be performed at this time. Following syndesmotic reduction and fixation, the ankle is plantarflexed in 15° and the FiberTape is passed through the eyelet of a 4.75-mm PEEK anchor. The location for the eyelet on the FiberTape is determined with the tip of the eyelet in the malleolar tunnel and a mark made at the level of the lower laser line. With tension on the graft and FiberTape , the two are sutured together at this location (**Fig. 7**) Insertion of the graft-tape construct is performed with the ankle in 15° of plantarflexion so that, with dorsiflexion and rollback of the talus, there will be tension on the graft in neutral position as in the native pDDL (**Fig. 8**). Once the posterior limb of the construct is in place, the ankle is dorsiflexed to neutral and a second tunnel is drilled into the talar footprint of the aDDL insertion, approximately 5 to 10 mm distal to the coronal plane location of the medial malleolar anchor. Another 4.75-mm anchor

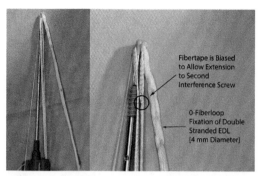

Fig. 6. Insertion device for the anchor combines a FiberTape (Arthrex) and an EDL tendon autograft that is approximately 4 mm in diameter. The tendon is secured with 0-FiberLoop suture (Arthrex) and passed through the anchor eyelet with the FiberTape. The tendon can be harvested locally proximal to the quadrification of the EDL tendon at the level of the inferior extensor retinaculum, usually with sufficient length to allow extension to the third interference screw. Note that the FiberTape is biased to gain maximal length to accommodate both limbs of the reconstruction.

is then placed in the same fashion. The ankle is placed in neutral and internal rotation position, keeping the hindfoot in valgus during implantation to maximize the resultant stability (**Fig. 9**). The authors no longer worry about overtensioning the graft or Fiber-Tape because our biomechanical testing has shown that creep does occur with this construct under physiologic cyclic loading, which is expected clinically with early motion. We have commonly found that the pDDL is intact and the aDDL alone requires reconstruction with syndesmosis reduction and repair (**Fig. 10**). The procedure can be modified by performing only the aDDL reconstruction (**Fig. 11**). We still follow the same order of preparing the syndesmosis repairs and then preparing the medial

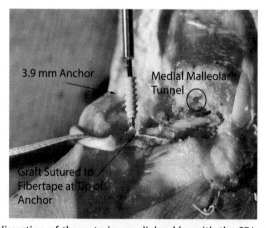

Fig. 7. Anatomic dissection of the anterior medial ankle, with the SDL reflected inferiorly. Once the posterior anchor with the graft-tape construct is secured to the talus, the Fiber-Tape (Arthrex) is measured in standard fashion to insert into a tunnel in the medial malleolus. The graft and tape are sutured together with parallel tension before insertion into the medial malleolar tunnel. The ankle is brought into 15° to 20° of plantarflexion to provide usual tension for the talus rollback with ankle dorsiflexion.

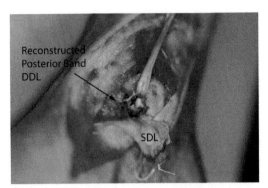

Fig. 8. Anatomic dissection of the anterior medial ankle, with the SDL reflected inferiorly, showing the final appearance of reconstruction of the posterior DDL fibers, with the limb for reconstruction of the anterior fibers retracted proximally. The posterior graft-tape construct is secured into the medial malleolus.

malleolar tunnel before completing the syndesmosis repairs. The medial malleolar and anterior talar anchor preparation and graft insertion are performed with the ankle in neutral, as described earlier. The SDL can then be repaired as described earlier. If a spring ligament reconstruction was also deemed necessary, an anterior limb of augmentation could be placed within the repair of the anterior SDL (see **Fig. 4**).

Postoperative Protocol

Splinting and non–weight bearing for 1 to 2 weeks is required to aid wound healing. Adjunctive procedures such as osteotomies may require longer protection; however, the preference is to stage these procedures in some patients in order to start early range of motion following the ligamentous repair. When reconstruction is limited to soft tissues, then active range of motion is begun after 1 to 2 weeks and progressive weight bearing in a removable cast boot that does not press on the incisions is begun.

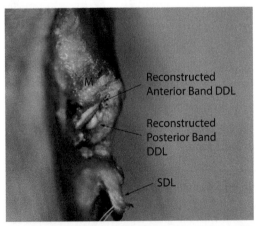

Fig. 9. Anatomic dissection of the anterior medial ankle, with the SDL reflected inferiorly, showing the reconstructed anterior band of the DDL secured in the talus in an anatomic coronal plane orientation. The SDL can be repaired to the medial malleolus (M), over the deep reconstruction.

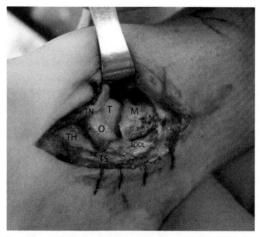

Fig. 10. Anatomic dissection of the anterior medial ankle showing the aDDL insufficiency after longitudinal division of the SDL in between the TN and TS fibers. The aDDL remnant has a fibrofatty appearance consistent with the failed healing response of an intra-articular ligament. The medial talar body (T) is dysmorphic with the absence of the normal fossa for insertion of the deep deltoid because the injury occurred when the patient was skeletally immature. The medial malleolus (M) is similarly dysmorphic without the normal flat surface for origin of the aDDL in the intercollicular fossa. There is an osteophyte ridge (O) of the medial talar body consistent with chronic medial instability. The talar head (TH) is seen distally.

Early mobilization with light band resistance exercises is advanced with physical therapy and, at 6 weeks, patients are fully weight bearing and transition to an ankle brace with progressive rehabilitation. Activities are limited to low-impact aerobics until 3 months and then progression to higher-impact activities can begin.

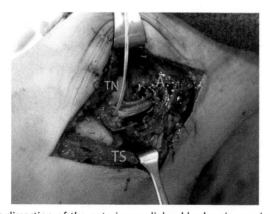

Fig. 11. Anatomic dissection of the anterior medial ankle showing an isolated reconstruction of the aDDL. The graft and tape have been inserted into the talus. The repair is then completed by suturing the TS component of the SDL to the talar insertion site with the attached #2 FiberWire (Arthrex). The TN band of the SDL (retracted superiorly) and the TS band are then repaired with a running 1.3-mm suture tape and the origin of the TN band is secured to the anterior medial malleolus with a small anchor (A).

SUMMARY AND FUTURE PERSPECTIVES

Deltoid ligament complex plays a crucial role in the overall stability of the ankle joint. CDI, or medial ankle instability, is a frequent injury that can develop following minor or major traumas of the foot and ankle, predominantly rotational injuries. CDI is frequently underdiagnosed or misdiagnosed, particularly when mild instability is present. Long-term residual instability can lead to PTOA. Adequate assessment of patients with suspected CDI is paramount, with identification of which deltoid ligament components (superficial and/or deep deltoid) are involved as well as the presence of combined syndesmotic and lateral ligament instability (multidirectional instability). Conservative treatment can be tried for stable or mildly unstable cases, but surgical treatment is usually the answer for the more severely unstable patients, as well as patients that fail conservative measures. Multiple surgical techniques for reconstruction of the different deltoid ligament components have been proposed in the literature, but very few in the setting of posttraumatic CDI and absence of associated progressive collapsing foot deformity. This article describes our preferred technique for reconstruction of the deep components of the deltoid ligament. Improved and optimized diagnostic tools for early and accurate diagnosis of subtle CDI are paramount. Low threshold for clinical diagnostic suspicion, in combination with static soft tissue (MRI) and dynamic bony advanced imaging (WBCT) can represent a potential game changer in the near future. Diagnostic, prospective, and comparative studies are needed to assess the different patterns of deltoid ligament injuries as well as the diverse repair/reconstruction techniques that can be used in the setting of posttraumatic CDI.

CLINICS CARE POINTS

- Chronic Deltoid Injuries/Instability (CDI) is frequently overlooked and under diagnosed.
- Undiagnosed/Untreated CDI represent one of the most important causes of Posttraumatic Osteoarthritis of the Ankle Joint.
- Identification of injuries/instability of specific bands of the superficial and deep deltoid ligaments, followed by adequate repair/reconstruction is paramount for improved outcomes.

DISCLOSURE

J.E. Femino: research support from Arthrex; paid consultant to Integra; unpaid consultant to OncoRegen. C. de Cesar Netto: paid consultant to Curvebeam, Ossio, Zimmer-Biomet, Nextremity, Paragon 28; stock options with Curvebeam; royalties from Paragon 28; media board member with Foot & Ankle International, treasurer for International WBCT Society, committee member for American Orthopaedic Foot & Ankle Society.

REFERENCES

1. Saltzman CL, Zimmerman MB, O'Rourke M, et al. Impact of comorbidities on the measurement of health in patients with ankle osteoarthritis. J Bone Joint Surg Am 2006;88(11):2366–72.

2. Glazebrook M, Daniels T, Younger A, et al. Comparison of health-related quality of life between patients with end-stage ankle and hip arthrosis. J Bone Joint Surg Am 2008;90(3):499–505.

3. Saltzman CL, Salamon ML, Blanchard GM, et al. Epidemiology of ankle arthritis: report of a consecutive series of 639 patients from a tertiary orthopaedic center. Iowa Orthop J 2005;25:44–6.

4. Alshalawi S, Galhoum AE, Alrashidi Y, et al. Medial ankle instability: the deltoid dilemma. Foot Ankle Clin 2018;23(4):639–57.

5. Hintermann B. Medial ankle instability. Foot Ankle Clin 2003;8(4):723–38.

6. Hintermann B, Valderrabano V, Boss A, et al. Medial ankle instability: an exploratory, prospective study of fifty-two cases. Am J Sports Med 2004;32(1):183–90.

7. Close JR. Some applications of the functional anatomy of the ankle joint. J Bone Joint Surg Am 1956;38-A(4):761–81.

8. Burns WC 2nd, Prakash K, Adelaar R, et al. Tibiotalar joint dynamics: indications for the syndesmotic screw–a cadaver study. Foot Ankle 1993;14(3):153–8.

9. Ramsey PL, Hamilton W. Changes in tibiotalar area of contact caused by lateral talar shift. J Bone Joint Surg Am 1976;58(3):356–7.

10. Campbell KJ, Michalski MP, Wilson KJ, et al. The ligament anatomy of the deltoid complex of the ankle: a qualitative and quantitative anatomical study. J Bone Joint Surg Am 2014;96(8):e62.

11. Savage-Elliott I, Murawski CD, Smyth NA, et al. The deltoid ligament: an in-depth review of anatomy, function, and treatment strategies. Knee Surg Sports Traumatol Arthrosc 2013;21(6):1316–27.

12. Takao M, Ozeki S, Oliva XM, et al. Strain pattern of each ligamentous band of the superficial deltoid ligament: a cadaver study. BMC Musculoskelet Disord 2020; 21(1):289.

13. Earll M, Wayne J, Brodrick C, et al. Contribution of the deltoid ligament to ankle joint contact characteristics: a cadaver study. Foot Ankle Int 1996;17(6):317–24.

14. Tochigi Y, Rudert MJ, Saltzman CL, et al. Contribution of articular surface geometry to ankle stabilization. J Bone Joint Surg Am 2006;88(12):2704–13.

15. Tochigi Y, Rudert MJ, Amendola A, et al. Tensile engagement of the peri-ankle ligaments in stance phase. Foot Ankle Int 2005;26(12):1067–73.

16. O'Loughlin PF, Murawski CD, Egan C, et al. Ankle instability in sports. Phys Sportsmed 2009;37(2):93–103.

17. Kofotolis ND, Kellis E, Vlachopoulos SP. Ankle sprain injuries and risk factors in amateur soccer players during a 2-year period. Am J Sports Med 2007;35(3): 458–66.

18. Waterman BR, Belmont PJ Jr, Cameron KL, et al. Epidemiology of ankle sprain at the United States Military Academy. Am J Sports Med 2010;38(4):797–803.

19. Buchhorn T, Sabeti-Aschraf M, Dlaska CE, et al. Combined medial and lateral anatomic ligament reconstruction for chronic rotational instability of the ankle. Foot Ankle Int 2011;32(12):1122–6.

20. Lauge-Hansen N. Ligamentous ankle fractures; diagnosis and treatment. Acta Chir Scand 1949;97(6):544–50.

21. Michelsen JD, Ahn UM, Helgemo SL. Motion of the ankle in a simulated supination-external rotation fracture model. J Bone Joint Surg Am 1996;78(7): 1024–31.

22. Goetz JE, Vasseenon T, Tochigi Y, et al. 3D talar kinematics during external rotation stress testing in hindfoot varus and valgus using a model of syndesmotic and deep deltoid instability. Foot Ankle Int 2019;40(7):826–35.

23. Murray MM, Martin SD, Martin TL, et al. Histological changes in the human anterior cruciate ligament after rupture. J Bone Joint Surg Am 2000;82(10):1387–97.
24. Sagi HC, Shah AR, Sanders RW. The functional consequence of syndesmotic joint malreduction at a minimum 2-year follow-up. J Orthop Trauma 2012;26(7): 439–43.
25. Weening B, Bhandari M. Predictors of functional outcome following transsyndesmotic screw fixation of ankle fractures. J Orthop Trauma 2005;19(2):102–8.
26. Ashraf A, Murphree J, Wait E, et al. Gravity stress radiographs and the effect of ankle position on deltoid ligament integrity and medial clear space measurements. J Orthop Trauma 2017;31(5):270–4.
27. Krahenbuhl N, Weinberg MW, Davidson NP, et al. Imaging in syndesmotic injury: a systematic literature review. Skeletal Radiol 2018;47(5):631–48.
28. Park SS, Kubiak EN, Egol KA, et al. Stress radiographs after ankle fracture: the effect of ankle position and deltoid ligament status on medial clear space measurements. J Orthop Trauma 2006;20(1):11–8.
29. Ovaska MT, Makinen TJ, Madanat R, et al. A comprehensive analysis of patients with malreduced ankle fractures undergoing re-operation. Int Orthop 2014; 38(1):83–8.
30. Lee S, Lin J, Hamid KS, et al. Deltoid Ligament Rupture in Ankle Fracture: Diagnosis and Management. J Am Acad Orthop Surg 2019;27(14):e648–58.
31. Stufkens SA, van den Bekerom MP, Kerkhoffs GM, et al. Long-term outcome after 1822 operatively treated ankle fractures: a systematic review of the literature. Injury 2011;42(2):119–27.
32. Valderrabano V, Horisberger M, Russell I, et al. Etiology of ankle osteoarthritis. Clin Orthop Relat Res 2009;467(7):1800–6.
33. Horisberger M, Valderrabano V, Hintermann B. Posttraumatic ankle osteoarthritis after ankle-related fractures. J Orthop Trauma 2009;23(1):60–7.
34. Crim J. Medial-sided Ankle Pain: Deltoid Ligament and Beyond. Magn Reson Imaging Clin N Am 2017;25(1):63–77.
35. Sman AD, Hiller CE, Refshauge KM. Diagnostic accuracy of clinical tests for diagnosis of ankle syndesmosis injury: a systematic review. Br J Sports Med 2013;47(10):620–8.
36. Stenquist DS, Miller C, Velasco B, et al. Medial tenderness revisited: Is medial ankle tenderness predictive of instability in isolated lateral malleolus fractures? Injury 2020;51(6):1392–6.
37. McGovern RP, Martin RL. Managing ankle ligament sprains and tears: current opinion. Open Access J Sports Med 2016;7:33–42.
38. Femino JE, Vaseenon T, Phisitkul P, et al. Varus external rotation stress test for radiographic detection of deep deltoid ligament disruption with and without syndesmotic disruption: a cadaveric study. Foot Ankle Int 2013;34(2):251–60.
39. Abdelaziz ME, Hagemeijer N, Guss D, et al. Evaluation of syndesmosis reduction on CT Scan. Foot Ankle Int 2019;40(9):1087–93.
40. Bhimani R, Ashkani-Esfahani S, Lubberts B, et al. Utility of volumetric measurement via weight-bearing computed tomography scan to diagnose syndesmotic instability. Foot Ankle Int 2020;41(7):859–65.
41. Burssens A, Vermue H, Barg A, et al. Templating of Syndesmotic Ankle Lesions by Use of 3D Analysis in Weightbearing and Nonweightbearing CT. Foot Ankle Int 2018;39(12):1487–96.
42. Del Rio A, Bewsher SM, Roshan-Zamir S, et al. Weightbearing cone-beam computed tomography of acute ankle syndesmosis injuries. J Foot Ankle Surg 2020;59(2):258–63.

43. Hagemeijer NC, Chang SH, Abdelaziz ME, et al. Range of normal and abnormal syndesmotic measurements using weightbearing CT. Foot Ankle Int 2019;40(12): 1430–7.

44. Shakoor D, Osgood GM, Brehler M, et al. Cone-beam CT measurements of distal tibio-fibular syndesmosis in asymptomatic uninjured ankles: does weight-bearing matter? Skeletal Radiol 2019;48(4):583–94.

45. Crim J, Longenecker LG. MRI and surgical findings in deltoid ligament tears. AJR Am J Roentgenol 2015;204(1):W63–9.

46. Dabash S, Elabd A, Potter E, et al. Adding deltoid ligament repair in ankle fracture treatment: Is it necessary? A systematic review. Foot Ankle Surg 2019;25(6): 714–20.

47. Wang X, Ma X, Zhang C, et al. Treatment of chronic deltoid ligament injury using suture anchors. Orthop Surg 2014;6(3):223–8.

48. Tennant JN, Rungprai C, Pizzimenti MA, et al. Risks to the blood supply of the talus with four methods of total ankle arthroplasty: a cadaveric injection study. J Bone Joint Surg Am 2014;96(5):395–402.

49. Bluman EM. Deltoid ligament injuries in ankle fractures: should I leave it or fix it? Foot Ankle Int 2012;33(3):236–8.

50. Butler BA, Hempen EC, Barbosa M, et al. Deltoid ligament repair reduces and stabilizes the talus in unstable ankle fractures. J Orthop 2020;17:87–90.

51. Lack W, Phisitkul P, Femino JE. Anatomic deltoid ligament repair with anchor-to-post suture reinforcement: technique tip. Iowa Orthop J 2012;32:227–30.

52. Mococain P, Bejarano-Pineda L, Glisson R, et al. Biomechanical Effect on Joint Stability of Including Deltoid Ligament Repair in an Ankle Fracture Soft Tissue Injury Model With Deltoid and Syndesmotic Disruption. Foot Ankle Int 2020. https://doi.org/10.1177/1071100720929007. 1071100720929007.

53. Salameh M, Alhammoud A, Alkhatib N, et al. Outcome of primary deltoid ligament repair in acute ankle fractures: a meta-analysis of comparative studies. Int Orthop 2020;44(2):341–7.

54. Woo SH, Bae SY, Chung HJ. Short-Term Results of a Ruptured Deltoid Ligament Repair During an Acute Ankle Fracture Fixation. Foot Ankle Int 2018;39(1):35–45.

55. Yu GR, Zhang MZ, Aiyer A, et al. Repair of the acute deltoid ligament complex rupture associated with ankle fractures: a multicenter clinical study. J Foot Ankle Surg 2015;54(2):198–202.

56. de Cesar Netto C, Deland JT, Ellis SJ. Guest editorial: expert consensus on adult-acquired flatfoot deformity. Foot Ankle Int 2020;41(10):1269–71.

57. Myerson MS, Thordarson DB, Johnson JE, et al. Classification and nomenclature: progressive collapsing foot deformity. Foot Ankle Int 2020;41(10):1271–6.

58. Brodell JD Jr, MacDonald A, Perkins JA, et al. Deltoid-Spring Ligament Reconstruction in Adult Acquired Flatfoot Deformity With Medial Peritalar Instability. Foot Ankle Int 2019;40(7):753–61.

59. Deland JT, de Asla RJ, Segal A. Reconstruction of the chronically failed deltoid ligament: a new technique. Foot Ankle Int 2004;25(11):795–9.

60. Deland JT, Ellis SJ, Day J, et al. Indications for deltoid and spring ligament reconstruction in progressive collapsing foot deformity. Foot Ankle Int 2020;41(10): 1302–6.

61. Ellis SJ, Williams BR, Wagshul AD, et al. Deltoid ligament reconstruction with peroneus longus autograft in flatfoot deformity. Foot Ankle Int 2010;31(9):781–9.

62. Fonseca LF, Baumfeld D, Mansur N, et al. Deltoid Insufficiency and Flatfoot—Oh Gosh, I'm Losing the Ankle! What Now? Tech Foot Ankle Surg 2019;18(4):202–7.

63. Jeng CL, Bluman EM, Myerson MS. Minimally invasive deltoid ligament reconstruction for stage IV flatfoot deformity. Foot Ankle Int 2011;32(1):21–30.
64. Lui TH. Technical tips: reconstruction of deep and superficial deltoid ligaments by peroneus longus tendon in stage 4 posterior tibial tendon dysfunction. Foot Ankle Surg 2014;20(4):295–7.
65. Nery C, Lemos A, Raduan F, et al. Combined spring and deltoid ligament repair in adult-acquired flatfoot. Foot Ankle Int 2018;39(8):903–7.
66. Oburu E, Myerson MS. Deltoid Ligament Repair in Flatfoot Deformity. Foot Ankle Clin 2017;22(3):503–14.
67. Jung HG, Park JT, Eom JS, et al. Reconstruction of superficial deltoid ligaments with allograft tendons in medial ankle instability: A technical report. Injury 2016; 47(3):780–3.
68. Pellegrini MJ, Torres N, Cuchacovich NR, et al. Chronic deltoid ligament insufficiency repair with Internal Brace augmentation. Foot Ankle Surg 2019;25(6): 812–8.
69. Hajewski CJ, Duchman K, Goetz J, et al. Anatomic Syndesmotic and Deltoid Ligament Reconstruction with Flexible Implants: A Technique Description. Iowa Orthop J 2019;39(1):21–7.
70. Guyton GP, DeFontes K 3rd, Barr CR, et al. Arthroscopic correlates of subtle syndesmotic injury. Foot Ankle Int 2017;38(5):502–6.

Current Trends in Treatment of Injuries to Spring Ligament

Caio Nery, MD, PhD[a,b,*], Daniel Baumfeld, MD, PhD[c]

KEYWORDS

- Spring ligament • Flatfoot • Deltoid ligament • Spring reconstruction

KEY POINTS

- It is important to diagnose spring ligament injuries because of the probable consequences if not treated.
- Flatfoot deformity and loss of correction of treated flatfoot are the consequences of neglected spring ligament repair or reconstruction.
- Direct repair of the spring ligament may only be suitable before the soft tissues become attenuated and degenerated.
- The combination of spring and deltoid injury is common, so reconstruction of both ligaments may be necessary.
- Spring ligament injury can occur in isolation in the absence of a tear of the posterior tibial tendon.

INTRODUCTION

Understanding of spring ligament injury has evolved as different patterns of insufficiency and injuries of this ligament and its consequences have been identified.[1]

The spring ligament is the main static supporter of the medial longitudinal arch, whereas the dynamic support is primarily guaranteed by the posterior tibial tendon (PTT). The deterioration of each of these supporting structures can result in a progressive collapsing foot deformity (PCFD).[2–4]

Identifying every detail of the pathophysiology of each condition in which these structures are involved is the key to an appropriate approach and treatment. Establishing the primary or secondary role of the spring ligament and other anatomy involved in the deformity and its response to trauma or chronic overload is essential

[a] Orthopedic & Traumatology Department, Federal University of São Paulo, Av. Albert Einstein, 627 – Morumbi, São Paulo, SP CEP 05652.000, Brazil; [b] Foot and Ankle Clinic; [c] Department of Locomotor Apparatus, Federal University of Minas Gerais, Av. Prof. Alfredo Balena, 190 - Belo Horizonte, MG CEP 30130-100, Brazil
* Corresponding author. Orthopedic & Traumatology Department, Federal University of São Paulo, Brazil.
E-mail address: caionerymd@gmail.com

Foot Ankle Clin N Am 26 (2021) 345–359
https://doi.org/10.1016/j.fcl.2021.03.008
1083-7515/21/© 2021 Elsevier Inc. All rights reserved.

for a perfect understanding of the process as a whole. Although chronic deterioration of the spring ligament can be found in the conventional setting of PCFD as a consequence of rupture of the PTT, it can also be the primary cause of that deformity, secondarily overloading all other structures.[1,2,5,6]

This article focuses on the new trends and options for repair and/or reconstruction of the spring ligament as a single unit and as part of PCFD.

THE PROBLEM

The spring ligament complex, together with the PTT, the plantar fascia, and the plantar ligaments, is an important stabilizer of the longitudinal arch of the foot. Even so, the importance of treating this ligament together with other bone and soft tissue reconstructions has not been totally elucidated.[7,8]

Although isolated reconstruction of the PTT was reported to yield a promising short-term outcome, long-term results were disappointing with a high failure rate.[9] Treatments were first centered only on the tendon and bone, but this deformity comprises far more than a ligament or tendon rupture or both because of the secondary changes and deformities that result. There is a high incidence (70%–80%) of attenuated or torn spring ligament in rupture of the PTT.[10] Extended procedures involving reconstruction of all associated lesions in adult-acquired flatfoot deformity, including the spring ligament, superficial deltoid, and bone stabilization, may lead to more normal biomechanics of the hindfoot and may result in more favorable clinical results.[11,12]

Because of the nature and function of most of the ligament structures of the talocalcaneonavicular joint (also called acetabulum pedis), the anatomic delimitation between them is difficult when not only artificial. For this reason, this article uses the term spring ligament complex to acknowledge the inability in determining the individual role and culpability of the superomedial and inferior calcaneonavicular ligaments together with the talonavicular fascicle of the superficial portion of the deltoid ligament in the physiology of stability as well as in the genesis of the imbalances in this region.

CLINICAL BACKGROUND AND DIAGNOSIS

It is impossible to accurately identify and differentiate each anatomic structure involved in the genesis of medial ankle instability. Because of its anatomic and functional origins, there are no clinical signs or specific maneuvers that are pathognomonic for each of the potentially injured ligaments. Clinical suspicion is increased when persistent medial midfoot pain is present with associated with pes planus, whether following trauma or not. Pain underneath the PTT more inferiorly located than over the course of the tendon, especially when resisted inversion is still present, is also a practical maneuver to enhance the diagnosis of spring ligament tear.

According to Hintermann,[13] patients may complain of the involved ankle giving way, especially in its medial face and in activities that require the external rotation of the leg while the foot is firmly on the ground (walking on even ground, downhill, or downstairs).[8,13] Tenderness over the medial surface of the ankle (medial gutter) and foot, especially during dorsiflexion of the ankle, and the positivity of the standing test are also important findings (**Fig. 1**).

The neutral heel push test, described by Pasapula and colleagues,[14] represents the first maneuver to clinically identify the involvement of the spring ligament in medial instability. The test is easy to perform by holding the hindfoot firmly with 1 hand while an abduction force is applied with the other hand at the medial surface of the first metatarsal. The test is considered negative when no movement can be detected with the maneuver, representing the integrity of the spring ligament complex. Any

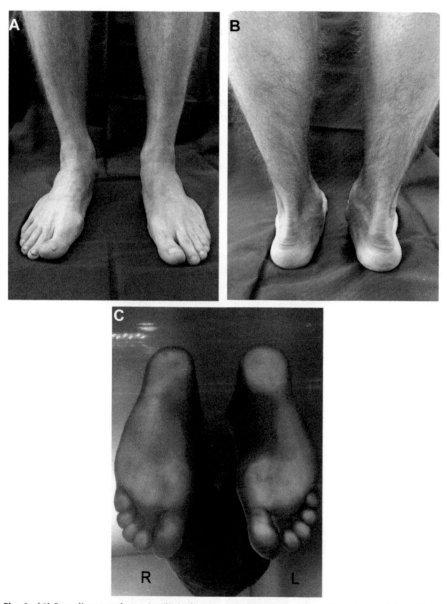

Fig. 1. (*A*) Standing test (anteriorclinical aspect). Subtle deformity of the affected foot (right in this patient), with valgus of the hindfoot and pronation of the foot as a whole. This condition can be corrected when the patient is asked to activate his posterior tendon muscle. (*B*) Standing test (posterior clinical aspect). Same patients as in (*A*) Bulging of the medial contour of the foot, slight heel valgus, and reduction of the medial longitudinal arch. The right foot is slightly pronated. (*C*) Podoscopy of the same patient as in (*A*) and (*B*). An important reduction of the plantar vault of the right foot can be confirmed through these plantar images, indicating the failure of the support structures of the medial longitudinal arch.

degree of translation of the forefoot, compared with the other foot, indicates a loss of integrity of the spring ligament complex (**Fig. 2**).[14]

Some investigators suggest that the presence of spring ligament injury is likely when midfoot abduction (>5° talar–first metatarsal angle and/or >30% talar head uncovering at weight-bearing anteroposterior [AP] view of the foot) and/or talonavicular sag (>−5° talar–first metatarsal angle at weight-bearing lateral view of the foot) are present on the plain weight-bearing radiographs.[14,15] Surgeons must be prepared to perform a repair or reconstruction of the spring ligament if confirmed during surgical inspection.

TRAUMATIC AND ISOLATED INJURIES

Acute isolated injuries of the spring ligament with normal tibialis posterior tendon have been infrequently diagnosed. Most patients had some type of sprain or minor twisting of the foot during walking or sport activity. The typical mechanism is forceful landing on a flatfoot, with some degree of eversion.[2,16] Isolated tears can also occur as a result of chronic attenuation in the absence of a PTT rupture, but this presentation is less common and more difficult to diagnose.

Spring ligament injuries are usually characterized by symptoms such as swelling along the bottom of the foot, deep aches, or pain and difficulty bearing weight on the foot. Failure to support the longitudinal arch may eventually result in adult-acquired flatfoot, or a fallen arch, with abduction of the midfoot.

Clinically, differentiation between isolated spring ligament and posterior tibialis tendon tear can be challenging. Patients may present as a tibialis posterior tendon rupture with history of trauma and a preserved function of the tendon. The tendon integrity and functionality can be tested during non–weight-bearing plantarflexion inversion of the foot or deformity correction during heel-rise test.[11,15]

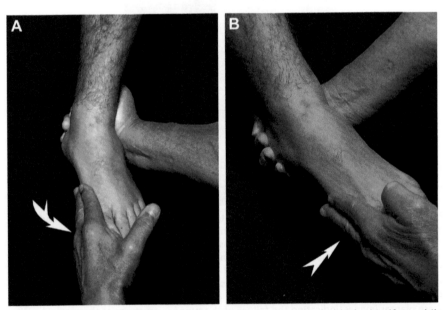

Fig. 2. (*A, B*) Neutral heel push test. With 1 hand, the examiner holds the hindfoot while applying an abduction force (*white arrow*) to the medial border of the forefoot with the other hand. The test is positive when any degree of translation of the forefoot is detected (compared with the other side).

Weight-bearing radiographs are mandatory. They can be initially normal or show different degrees of talonavicular subluxation and talus drop (**Fig. 3**).

MRI can be helpful to enhance the diagnose. Toye and colleagues[17] correlated surgically proven spring ligament tears with MRI findings: abnormal spring ligament caliber, signal intensity, waviness, full-thickness gap, and posterior tibial tendinopathy. The finding unique to cases with surgically proven tears is a full-thickness gap in the ligament.[18,19]

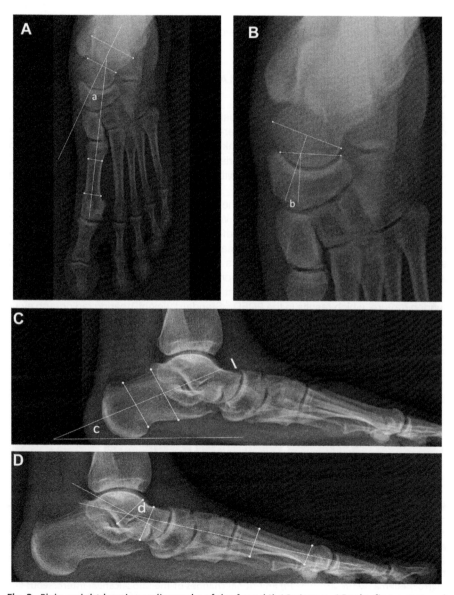

Fig. 3. Plain weight-bearing radiographs of the foot. (*A*) AP view: a, AP talo–first metatarsal angle. (*B*) AP view (closeup): b, talus coverage angle. (*C*) Lateral view (*detail*): c, calcaneal pitch angle. (*D*) Lateral view: d, Meary angle.

The authors use MRI almost routinely. This imaging examination helps to clarify the clinical diagnosis and prepare the surgical treatment when indicated.

MRI can also present[20]:

- Bone bruising of medial/plantar aspects of talar head-neck, sustentaculum, and anterior process of calcaneus and lateral navicular (consistent with midfoot injury).
- High-grade tear of superomedial portion of spring ligament and tibiospring component of superficial deltoid ligament. Bands of the spring ligament thickened/scarred.
- Partial tearing of the cervical and interosseous talocalcaneal ligaments in the sinus tarsi (**Fig. 4**).

ASSOCIATED INJURIES (PROGRESSIVE COLLAPSING FLATFOOT DEFORMITY AND/OR OTHER CHRONIC INJURIES)

PCFD is primarily caused by spring ligament rupture and tibialis posterior (TP) dysfunction and a consequence of degenerative tendon failure or rupture. Initially, patients may present with medial foot and ankle pain, swelling, and mild weakness, with almost no deformity. The single-limb heel rise can be painful or impossible to achieve. As the disease evolves, a flexible PCFD with a significant PTT attenuation or rupture can be associated.

The deformity consists of flattening of the medial longitudinal arch, hindfoot valgus, forefoot abduction, and forefoot varus. With progression, patients are unable to perform a single-limb heel rise, but the hindfoot remains flexible. In later stages, deformity can be rigid and joint degeneration can be also present. Myerson[21] introduced stage IV of flat foot disease, which occurs when the talus tilts into valgus within the ankle mortise secondary to deltoid and spring ligament rupture.[11,13,21] Furthermore, spring ligament deficiency is often present but not specifically tested clinically in TP tendon rupture, which results in the PCFD.[2] Standard weight-bearing radiograph evaluation does not differ from the typical characteristics described for PTT rupture: radiological signs of medial arch collapse and progressive subluxation of the talonavicular joint in both coronal and sagittal planes can be found.

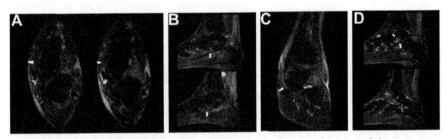

Fig. 4. (A) MRI of a patient with foot pronation trauma. showing thinning of the superomedial component of the spring ligament (*white arrow*) and complete rupture of the superomedial component of the spring ligament (*white arrowhead*). (B) Hypersignal in the anatomic area corresponding with the inferomedial portion of the spring ligament with signs of complete rupture of this component (*white arrows*). (C) The white arrow points to the rupture area of the superomedial component of the spring ligament. (D) Bone marrow edema (*white arrowhead*) and signal changes of the talocalcaneal interosseous ligament (*white arrow*) in the same patient as in (A–C). Hypersignal of the talocalcaneal interosseous ligament (*gray arrowhead*) and calcaneal bone cysts (*gray arrow*) of the same patient.

The diagnosis mostly depends on MRI evaluation and direct intraoperative inspection. The sensitivity of spring ligament tear on MRI is reported to range from 55% to 77%, whereas specificity is almost 100%.[10]

MRI findings consistent with spring ligament tears include increased signal changes on T2-weighted sequences associated with thickening (>5 mm) or thinning (<2 mm) of the spring ligament.

Deland and colleagues[10] analyzed high-resolution MRI studies in patients with flatfoot deformities. They found the PTT to be pathologic in 100% of the patients; the superomedial component of the spring ligament in 87%; the inferior component of the spring ligament in 74%; the talocalcaneal interosseous ligament in 48%; and the anterior superficial deltoid, the deep deltoid, and the posterior superficial deltoid in 33%.[10]

REPAIR OR RECONSTRUCT

Avascularity of the central part of the superomedial portion of the spring ligament could be a predisposing factor for these ligament injuries, acute or chronic. Also, the native fibrocartilaginous origin of this ligament may lead to progressive attenuation and degeneration when overloading of the talonavicular joint occurs. As a consequence, it becomes incapable of holding load.[15,22,23]

Surgeons can conjecture about the degree of injury of the spring ligament through the amount of the talar head protrusion or subluxation. Mild fraying or weakening, without a gross tear, may present with less midfoot abduction. Partial to complete tear of the spring ligament is often associated with talar head uncovered with medial protrusion and progressive abduction.

The mechanism of injury, the amount of possible soft tissue healing, and the clinical findings help surgeons to choose between direct repair, repair with protection (augmentation), or reconstruction.

Direct repair of the spring ligament may only be suitable before the soft tissues become attenuated and degenerated[6,24]:

- Traumatic injuries without history of chronic flatfoot, without signs of degeneration, with normal radiograph and positive MRI.

When the authors are facing an patient with PCFD with PTT and spring ligament rupture, often the result is a chronic degenerative process, in which the native tissues become attenuated and unable to heal or even to be repaired. In those cases, augmentation or reconstruction of the spring ligament complex is favored rather than direct repair.[25] Patients in this situation may present a clear clinical status with more valgus and abduction. Radiography often shows a sag at the talonavicular joint and the talus head is grossly uncovered in weight-bearing AP view. In such cases, a tendon graft can be used to reconstruct the spring ligament and can also be augmented with sutures or high-mechanical-resistance tapes.[1,24]

TREATMENT

When dealing with a patient for spring ligament surgical treatment, the only additional concern is a clear and detailed surgical plan to ensure the availability of all the resources to reconstruct or repair the ligament. In the setting of PCFD, the protective/corrective hindfoot osteotomies and tendon transfers should be planned and performed as usual. These procedures are not discussed in this article.

The need for a spring ligament reconstruction can be confirmed fluoroscopically showing incomplete correction of talonavicular abduction after lateral column lengthening of other hindfoot procedures. In clinical practice, it is unlikely to encounter a patient who is candidate for a lateral column lengthening without a spring ligament tear. However, is common to see surgeons performing lateral column procedures without any approach to this ligament. The authors' algorithm relies on combinations of calcaneal osteotomy, and medical procedures, including tendon transfer and ligament reconstruction.

DIRECT REPAIR

Spring ligament direct repair is preferable for acute lesions without degeneration, but this ligament tear is frequently a result of a chronic degenerative process, leading to an attenuation of the tissue, which makes repairing it unpredictable.[2,18,24,25]

Direct repair can be performed through medial incision, as used for PTT debridement and/or tendon transfers.

Some techniques have been proposed:

- Resecting the lesions ends and suturing the remaining portions with stiches.
- Advancement and reinsertion of the ligament through transosseous navicular drill holes, plication of the talonavicular articular capsule, and retensioning in the vest-over-pants fashion (**Fig. 5**).[26,27]
- Endoscopic technique, described by Lui,[28] for repairing the superficial deltoid ligament and the spring ligament complex. Repair is performed through a PTT endoscopy and/or talonavicular arthroscopy. This technique provides limited soft tissue dissection. Surgical tightening of the ligament through a wedge resection or reefing has been described; however, with an attenuated ligament, these repairs are often tenuous.

REPAIR WITH INTERNAL BRACE

The InternalBrace FiberTape ligament augmentation device (Arthrex, Naples, FL) has been reported in a clinical series as an adjunct for spring ligament augmentation for the treatment of flatfoot correction with excellent clinical results at short-term follow-up.[26,29] Furthermore, this device has been safe and effective when used to augment lateral ligament repairs, and allows accelerated rehabilitation and recovery.[30] In addition, it has been studied biomechanically for this indication and has shown improved strength compared with standard ligament repair.[31] The use of the Fiber-Tape device to augment spring ligament repair may have mechanical benefits under cyclic loading, especially at higher load magnitudes. The idea of this concept is to help to stabilize and protect the soft tissues during the healing process.

The procedure is performed as follows:

- After a careful dissection in which all the deteriorated tissue is resected, the remnant spring ligament is repaired with an imbrication suture, and a tendon transfer, usually the flexor digitorum longus (FDL), is prepared.
- Protection of the local soft tissue repair with the internal brace concept using the FiberTape starts with the insertion of a 4.75 × 15-mm SwiveLock (Arthrex Inc, Naples, FL) with FiberTape suture at the medial surface of the sustentaculum tali.
- Both bands of the FiberTape attached to the sustentaculum tali are passed through the bone tunnel of the navicular: 1 from dorsal to plantar and the other, together with the FDL tendon, from plantar to dorsal. Both FiberTape suture bands aimed to rebuild and protect the spring ligament superomedial and inferomedial portions.

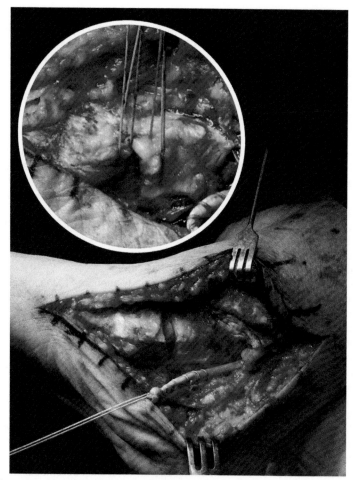

Fig. 5. The area of rupture of the spring ligament that has already been debrided and that results in a failure with exposure of the talar head. Detail shows the rupture area being tensioned and sutured to restore local stability.

- Once the proper tensioning of both FiberTape suture limbs and the FDL tendon is achieved, a Bio-Tenodesis screw (Arthrex Inc, Naples, FL) is inserted from plantar to dorsal, stabilizing the construct.

The internal brace concept can also be used to repair isolated tears. The spring ligament can be reconstructed with any type of graft (allograft or autograft) and then the fiber tape can add to the graft to reinforce it. This technique may enhance the strength of the reconstruction and may allow the tissues to heal without any lengthening during the postoperative period.

SPRING AND DELTOID LIGAMENT–ASSOCIATED LESIONS

The authors currently perform reconstruction of both ligaments in association because in, our experience the combination of spring and deltoid ligament injury is common, especially the superficial band. The understanding of the closely related anatomy of the spring ligament and the deltoid complex led us to describe a reconstruction technique in this field. The superficial deltoid ligament blends into the spring ligament, making a confluent ligament area in the distal superficial deltoid insertion.[29]

One reason for this approach is that both ligaments provide static stability to the talar head and hence to the talonavicular joint. Moreover, is thought that they can support the medial longitudinal arch and provide kinetic coupling between the ankle, hindfoot, and the forefoot.[15]

The technique to reconstruct both ligaments is as follows:

- The first step of the ligament repair uses the remaining local tissue of the deltoid and spring ligament with an imbrication suture as described earlier in this article.
- Protection of the local soft tissue repair with the internal brace concept using the FiberTape started with the insertion of a 4.75 × 15-mm SwiveLock (Arthrex Inc, Naples, FL) with FiberTape suture at the intercollicular groove region of the medial malleolus (**Fig. 6**A).
- A second bone tunnel is drilled at the talar neck, and a new 4.75 × 15-mm SwiveLock anchors 1 arm band of the FiberTape already attached to the medial malleolus, reconstructing the anterior tibiotalar component of the deltoid ligament (**Fig. 6**B).
- The second band of the FiberTape that is already anchored to the medial malleolus is passed through the 4-mm PEEK eyelet of a 4.75 × 15-mm SwiveLock in which another #2 FiberTape is mounted.
- After making a bone hole at the medial surface of the sustentaculum tali using the appropriate drill bit (**Fig. 6**C), the double-loaded SwiveLock anchor is introduced, repairing the tibiocalcaneal segment of the deltoid ligament (**Fig. 6**D).
- It is important to obtain an adequate tensioning of the FiberTape by making the measurements and sliding the end of the application instrument according to the manufacturer's instructions (see **Fig. 6**D). At that time, the foot should be kept in a neutral position, avoiding overcorrection.
- As the last step of the procedure, both bands of the FiberTape attached to the sustentaculum tali are passed through a bone tunnel at the navicular: 1 from dorsal to plantar and the other from plantar to dorsal (**Fig. 6**E). Both FiberTape suture bands are intended to augment both (superomedial and inferomedial) portions of the spring ligament.
- Once the proper tensioning of both FiberTape suture limbs is achieved, a Bio-Tenodesis Screw (Arthrex Inc, Naples, FL) or a 4.75 × 15-mm SwiveLock anchor is inserted from plantar to dorsal, stabilizing the construct (**Fig. 6**F).
- As a final step of medial ligament repair and augmentation, the superficial layers of the ligament area together with the retinaculum can be retensioned and fixed with the sutures that come from the anchors used, creating a homogeneous and safe aspect (**Fig. 6**G, H).

RECONSTRUCTION OF THE SPRING LIGAMENT

Several options have been described to reconstruct the spring ligament, most of them in cadaveric studies or small case series using the superficial deltoid ligament, peroneus longus tendon, split anterior tibial tendon, flexor hallucis longus tendon, or allografts.[8,32–34]

Although tendon harvest is associated with some degree of patient morbidity and loss of strength, reconstruction with tendon autograft could, theoretically, support load and forces at the talonavicular joint and possibly maintain correction of the deformity better than direct repair.

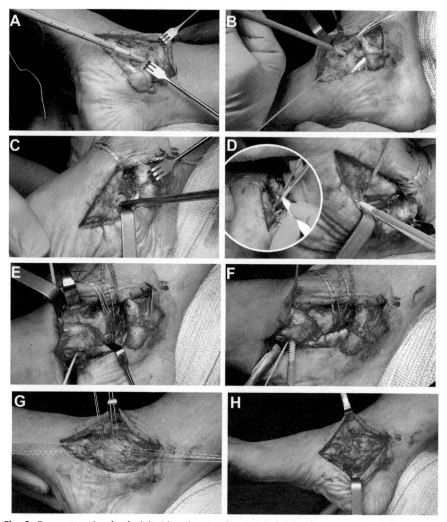

Fig. 6. Reconstructing both deltoid and spring ligament. (*A*) Anchor mounted with a tape at the intercolicular groove. (*B*)Reconstructing the anterior tibiotalar ligament. (*C*) Preparing the anchorage at the sustentaculum tali. (*D*) Reconstructing the tibiocalcaneal ligament (note the double loaded anchor). (*E*) Reconstructing the spring ligament. (*F*) After proper tensioning a bioteonodesis screw is introduced at the navicular bone tunnel. (*G*) Reattaching the soft tissue over the reconstructed ligament structures. (*H*) The final aspect of the construct.

Advantages and disadvantages of each procedure to reconstruct the spring ligament are related to graft harvest, bone tunnel position, and availability of implant fixation. The literature does not offer definitive information to help surgeons to choose the best or the most reliable technique to reconstruct this ligament.

Decision-making concerns related to the reconstruction of the spring ligament[18,35–39]:

- Anatomic or nonanatomic reconstructions
- Bone tunnels

- Choice of graft: allograft or autograft
- Choice of implant tendon to bone anchor fixation, buttress screw, bone tunnels, biotenodesis screws

Anatomic reconstruction

- Superior to plantar bone tunnel at the navicular bone, medial to lateral tunnel at the sustentaculum tali
- Graft is passed thought the navicular bone and the 2 remaining limbs are fixed at the sustentaculum tali

Nonanatomic reconstruction

- Navicular bone to the medial malleolus
- Navicular bone to medial malleolus and medial malleolus to calcaneus bone
- Deltoid ligament bone block graft from the medial malleolus to the navicular bone
- Peroneus tendon transfer from lateral to medial
- Flexor hallux longus from plantar to medial

POSTOPERATIVE CARE

Postoperatively, patients should be immobilized in a short-leg splint for at least 2 weeks until sutures are removed. After this, a transition to a non–weight-bearing boot for an additional 4 weeks is recommended. At 6 to 8 weeks postoperatively, patients may begin physiotherapy with weight bearing as tolerated in a removable walker boot.

SUMMARY

The spring ligament has been elucidated as the main static restraint of the talonavicular joint.[4] These ligament injuries are one of the causes of midfoot abduction deformity and loss of the medial arch of the foot. Spring ligament complex lesions are generally secondary to PTT rupture. Chronic overload during the midstance and heel-rise phase of the gait result in attenuation and tearing of the spring ligament complex, which is commonly found in flexible PCFD. This ligament is elongated in more than 87% of these patients. Acute injuries can also occur, but are rare.[2,40]

Physicians can detect laxity and/or insufficiency of the spring ligament by a simple clinical test, known as the neutral heel lateral push test. A cadaveric study validated this test, showing its ability to detect spring ligament rupture in isolation of PTT rupture.[12] Diagnosis can also be enhanced with MRI, with images showing a thickness greater than 5 mm and signal heterogeneity as criteria for an abnormal spring ligament. In the literature, MRI shows an acceptable sensitivity and specificity for detecting an abnormal spring ligament of 83% and 79%, respectively.[15,41]

Most of the studies in the literature on spring ligament reconstruction have been limited to level IV evidence and expert opinions. Even so, there is growing interest among orthopedic surgeons in including spring ligament repair or reconstruction as part of the flatfoot treatment plan because bony procedures and tendon transfers alone commonly fail to reestablishment the midfoot arch in long-term follow-up. Some evidence suggests that ligament reconstruction is capable of providing an excellent correction of the talonavicular deformity when performed in combination with tendon transfers and osteotomies.[2,6,11,15,27,42,43] Nevertheless, comparative clinical studies with patient-reported outcomes are necessary to quantify the real effect of these techniques.

Until now there has been little published evidence available on the clinical outcomes of spring ligament reconstruction with a synthetic ligament,[27] although biomechanical studies have shown that FiberTape is durable enough for cycle loading under simulated weight bearing.[31] A recent article compared 17 spring ligament reconstructions using synthetic ligament augmentation with 16 reconstruction using hamstring allograft.[37] There were improvements in radiological alignment in both groups; however, superior patient-reported outcomes were found in the synthetic ligament group.

The efficacy of such techniques has been difficult to quantify because of variable approaches and the number of concomitant procedures performed during flatfoot reconstruction.

In conclusion, the authors believe is important to diagnose spring ligament injuries because of the probable consequences if not treated, such as acquired flatfoot deformity and loss of correction of treated flatfoot. Surgical treatment is indicated according to patient clinical findings and the type of ligament injury.

CLINICS CARE POINT

- This article presents an overview of the updated data on the treatment option for the spring ligament injuries.

REFERENCES

1. Tryfonidis M, Jackson W, Mansour R, et al. Acquired adult flat foot due to isolated plantar calcaneonavicular (spring) ligament insufficiency with a normal tibialis posterior tendon. Foot Ankle Surg 2008;14(2):89–95.
2. Masaragian HJ, Ricchetti HO, Testa C. Acute Isolated Rupture of the Spring Ligament. Foot Ankle Int 2013;34(1):150–4.
3. Amaha K, Nimura A, Yamaguchi R, et al. Anatomic study of the medial side of the ankle base on the joint capsule: an alternative description of the deltoid and spring ligament. J Exp Orthop 2019;6(1):2–9.
4. Richie DH Jr. Biomechanics and clinical analysis of the adult acquired flatfoot. Clin Podiatric Med Surg 2007;24(4):617–44.
5. Deland JT. Spring ligament complex and flatfoot deformity: curse or blessing? Foot Ankle Int 2012;33(3):239–43.
6. Patel M, barbosa M, Kadakia AR. Role of Spring and Deltoid Ligament Reconstruction for Adult Acquired Flatfoot Deformity. Tech Foot Ankle 2017;16:124–35.
7. Taniguchi A, Tanaka Y, Takakura Y, et al. Anatomy of the spring ligament. J Bone Joint Surgery Am 2003;85(11):2174–8.
8. Alshalawi S, Galhoum AE, Alrashidi Y, et al. Medial ankle instability : the deltoid dilemma. Foot Ankle Clin North Am 2018;1–19. https://doi.org/10.1016/j.fcl.2018.07.008.
9. Pinney SJ, Lin SS. Current concept review: acquired adult flatfoot deformity. Foot Ankle Int 2006;27(1):1–10.
10. Deland JT, de Asla RJ, Sung I-H, et al. Posterior tibial tendon insufficiency: which ligaments are involved? Foot Ankle Int 2005;26(6):427–35.
11. Brodell JD Jr, MacDonald A, Perkins JA, et al. Deltoid-spring ligament reconstruction in adult acquired flatfoot deformity with medial peritalar instability. Foot Ankle Int 2019;40(7):753–61.
12. Smith JT, Bluman EM. Update on stage IV acquired adult flatfoot disorder. Foot Ankle Clin 2012;17(2):351–60.
13. Hintermann B. Medial ankle instability. Foot Ankle Clin N Am 2003;8(4):723–38.

14. Pasapula C, Devany A, Magan A, et al. Neutral heel lateral push test: The first clinical examination of spring ligament integrity. Foot 2015;25(2):69–74.

15. Bastias GF, Dalmau-Pasto M, Astudillo C, et al. Spring ligament instability. Foot Ankle Clin North Am 2018;1–20. https://doi.org/10.1016/j.fcl.2018.07.012.

16. Weerts B, Warmerdam PE, Faber FWM. Isolated spring ligament rupture causing acute flatfoot deformity: case report. Foot Ankle Int 2012;33(2):148–50.

17. Toye LR, Helms CA, Hoffman BD, et al. MRI of Spring Ligament Tears. AJR 2005; 184:1475–80.

18. Vadell AM, Peratta M. Calcaneonavicular Ligament : anatomy, diagnosis and treatment. Foot Ankle Clin N Am 2012;17(3):437–48.

19. Crim JR, Beals TC, Nickisch F, et al. Deltoid ligament abnormalities in chronic lateral ankle instability. Foot Ankle Int 2011;32(9):873–8.

20. Mengiardi B, Pinto C, Zanetti M. Spring ligament complex and posterior tibial tendon: mr anatomy and findings in acquired adult flatfoot deformity. Semin Musculoskelet Radiol 2016;20(01):104–15.

21. Myerson MS. Adult acquired flatfoot deformity: treatment of dysfunction of the posterior tibial tendon. Instr Course Lect 1997;46:393–405.

22. Domzalski M, Kwapisz A, Zabierek S. Morphology of Spring Ligament Fibrocartilage Complex Lesions. J Am Podiatric Med Assoc 2019;109(5):1–5.

23. Benjamin M, Ralphs JR. Fibrocartilage in tendons and ligaments - an adaptation to compressive load. J Anat 1998;193(4):481–94.

24. Orr JD, Nunley JA. Isolated spring ligament failure as a cause of adult-acquired flatfoot deformity. Foot Ankle Int 2013;34(6):818–23.

25. Deland JT. The adult acquired flatfoot and spring ligament complex: Pathology and implications for treatment. Foot Ankle Clin N Am 2001;6(1):129–35.

26. Acevedo J, Vora A. Anatomical Reconstruction of the Spring Ligament Complex. Foot Ankle Spec 2013;6(6):441–5.

27. Steginsky B, Vora A. What to do with the spring ligament. Foot Ankle Clin North Am 2017;1–13. https://doi.org/10.1016/j.fcl.2017.04.005.

28. Lui TH. Endoscopic repair of the superficial deltoid ligament and spring ligament. Arthrosc Tech 2016;5(3):e621–5.

29. Nery C, Lemos AVKC, Raduan F, et al. Combined spring and deltoid ligament repair in adult-acquired flatfoot. Foot Ankle Int 2018;39(8):903–7.

30. Kerkhoffs G, Van Dijk N. Acute lateral ankle ligament ruptures in the athlete. FCL 2013;18(2):215–8.

31. Aynardi MC, Saloky K, Roush EP, et al. Biomechanical evaluation of spring ligament augmentation with the fibertape device in a cadaveric flatfoot model. Foot Ankle Int 2019;40(5):596–602.

32. Ryssman DB, Jeng CL. Reconstruction of the spring ligament with a posterior tibial tendon autograft: technique tip. Foot Ankle Int 2017;38(4):452–6.

33. Palmanovich E, Shabat S, Brin YS, et al. Novel reconstruction technique for an isolated plantar calcaneonavicular (SPRING) ligament tear: A 5 case series report. Foot 2017;30:1–4.

34. Ellis SJ, Williams BR, Wagshul AD, et al. Deltoid Ligament Reconstruction with Peroneus Longus Autograft in Flatfoot Deformity. Foot Ankle Int 2010;31(09): 781–9.

35. Palmanovich E, Shabat S, Brin YS, et al. Anatomic Reconstruction Technique for a Plantar Calcaneonavicular (Spring) Ligament Tear. J Foot Ankle Surg 2015;54(6): 1124–6.

36. Mousavian A, Orapin J, Chinanuvathana A, et al. Anatomic spring ligament and posterior tibial tendon reconstruction: new concept of double bundle PTT and a novel technique for spring ligament. Arch Bone Joint Surg 2017;5(3):201–5.

37. Heyes G, Swanton E, Vosoughi AR, et al. Comparative study of spring ligament reconstructions using either hamstring allograft or synthetic ligament augmentation. Foot Ankle Int 2020. https://doi.org/10.1177/1071100720917375. 1071100720917375.

38. Grunfeld R, Oh I, Flemister S, et al. Reconstruction of the Deltoid-Spring Ligament: Tibiocalcaneonavicular Ligament Complex. Tech Foot Ankle Surg 2016; 15(1):39–45.

39. Fonseca L, Baumfeld D, Nery C, et al. Deltoid insufficiency and flatfoot—oh gosh, i'm losing the ankle! what now? Tech Foot Ankle Surg 2019;18(4):202–7.

40. Cromeens BP, Kirchhoff CA, Patterson RM, et al. An attachment-based description of the medial collateral and spring ligament complexes. Foot Ankle Int 2015; 36(6):710–21.

41. Crim J. MR imaging evaluation of subtle lisfranc injuries: the midfoot sprain. Magn Reson Imaging Clin North Am 2008;16(1):19–27.

42. Masaragian HJ, Massetti S, Perin F, et al. Flatfoot deformity due to isolated spring ligament injury. J Foot Ankle Surg 2020;1–10. https://doi.org/10.1053/j.jfas.2019. 09.011.

43. Ribbans WJ, Garde A. Tibialis posterior tendon and deltoid and spring ligament injuries in the elite athlete. Foot Ankle Clin North Am 2013;18(2):255–91.

Deltoid Rupture in Ankle Fractures

To Repair or Not to Repair?

Jan Joost I. Wiegerinck, MD, PhD[a], Sjoerd A. Stufkens, MD, PhD[b],*

KEYWORDS

- Deltoid • Ankle • Fracture • Rupture • Medial • Ligament • Instability

KEY POINTS

- The deltoid ligament plays a key role in ankle fracture treatment.
- Superiority of suturing the deltoid ligament in all ruptures is not proven.
- There may be additional advantage of deltoid ligament repair in cases of deltoid and syndesmotic insufficiency.

INTRODUCTION

Deltoid ligament ruptures are seen in all shapes and sizes. In ankle fractures, a deep deltoid ligament rupture is the equivalent of a medial malleolus fracture. It usually renders the ankle joint unstable[1] and is therefore in most cases an indication for surgery: open reduction and internal fixation of the fibula fracture and in some cases fixation of the posterior malleolus or placement of syndesmotic screws.[2,3] If the deltoid ligament is partially ruptured, the ankle joint might be stable or unstable. Sometimes there is a combination of a medial malleolus (anterior colliculus) avulsion fracture and a deep deltoid ligament rupture.[4]

Historically, there have been several steps in the evolution of understanding of ankle fractures. Maisonneuve, Danis, Weber, Lauge-Hansen and many others contributed greatly, and their names are forever bound to ankle fractures.[5] Understanding the biomechanics of ankle fractures helps to predict which parts are osseous and which parts are ligamentous injuries.[6] The importance of the deltoid ligament in ankle fractures has been subject to many investigations. To diagnose a deltoid ligament injury correctly is of paramount importance. Conservative treatment of unstable fractures renders poor outcomes compared with operative treatment.[7] The failure of

Funded by: VSNU2020.
^a Bergman Clinics, Braillelaan 10, Rijswijk 2289 CM, The Netherlands; ^b Amsterdam University Medical Centers, Location AMC, Meibergdreef 9, Amsterdam 1105 AZ, The Netherlands
* Corresponding author.
E-mail address: s.a.stufkens@amsterdamumc.nl

Foot Ankle Clin N Am 26 (2021) 361–371
https://doi.org/10.1016/j.fcl.2021.03.009
1083-7515/21/© 2021 The Author(s). Published by Elsevier Inc.
foot.theclinics.com

conservative treatment of supposedly stable ankle fractures is probably caused by the misdiagnosed medial injury.[8]

The authors consider recognizing and understanding instability of the bimalleolar and trimalleolar ankle fractures the first priority. This article addresses the question of which acutely ruptured deltoid ligaments that are part of an ankle fracture could benefit from suturing in order to help restore ankle stability.

EPIDEMIOLOGY

Supination external rotation is the mechanism that causes approximately 80% of all ankle fractures. The frequency of injury to the deltoid ligament in supination external rotation fractures is higher than previously expected.[9,10] In 20% of Weber B–type fractures, the deltoid ligament is ruptured, and in 36% of Weber C–type fractures.[11] The most common injury mechanism for ankle fractures with concomitant deltoid ligament injury is a supination external rotation type 4 trauma according to the Lauge-Hansen classification. The mechanisms underlying supination external rotation and pronation external rotation fractures are similar. The difference is the position of the foot at the moment of external rotation. With a foot in pronation, there is initial tension on the medial structures. A lateral fracture resulting from pronation external rotation is unstable because there is always a medial fracture or deltoid rupture. Moreover, Rasmussen and colleagues[12] found that the deep portions of the deltoid ligament in particular, which are thought to be the main stabilizers, could rupture in external rotation, whereas the superficial components remain intact.

DIAGNOSIS AND IMAGING

In the acute setting, malalignment, ecchymosis, and profound edema of the affected ankle can be found. It has been shown that clinical examination is a poor indicator for deltoid ligament injury, with an accuracy of 42%,[13] so additional diagnostics are often a necessity. This finding is related to the specific portion of the deltoid that is injured: when clinical symptoms are present, it may be likely that there is a soft tissue injury. This injury could consist of only the superficial deltoid ligaments with intact deep structures. The superficial ligaments provide a minor contribution to the medial stability of the ankle. The deep deltoid often ruptures off the medial aspect of the talus, and the superficial deltoid usually ruptures off the anterior distal tibia. Additional diagnostics primarily consist of conventional imaging focusing on the medial clear space (MCS) where widening can be found; 4 mm in a nonstressed mortise view and/or a superior tibiotalar clear space greater than 1 mm are considered pathologic. Moreover, normal values are reported to vary from 1 to 5 mm.[14] An MCS of more than 4 mm, with that value being at least 1 mm greater than the superior tibiotalar space, is accepted to represent a deep deltoid ligament rupture. On stressed mortise views, an MCS greater than 5 mm is considered pathologic.[14] Indications for surgery have been an MCS greater than 4 mm, MCS 1 mm or greater than the superior tibiotalar clear space, or any lateral talar shift seen perioperatively after fracture fixation. Ultrasonography is a promising modality, with up to 100% sensitivity and specificity reported,[15,16] but is often difficult to incorporate in an emergency department setting because of its time-consuming nature and the expertise required. MRI is considered by many to be the gold standard,[17,18] but also has not found its way into standard emergency ankle fracture care because of the high costs. There has been no level 1 study performed assessing the role of ultrasonography and/or MRI in the initial diagnostic pathway of ankle fractures. Intraoperatively, the diagnosis of a deltoid ligament rupture can be made by manual stress testing under fluoroscopy, or with a hook

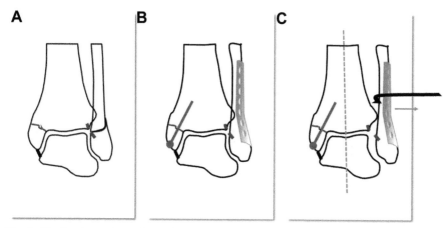

Fig. 1. The hook test is used mainly to test syndesmotic stability. (*A*) A typical trimalleolar fracture with a medial malleolus fracture, intact deltoid, and a Weber B–type fibula fracture. (*B*) After medial malleolus fixation, the talus is held underneath the talus. After fibula fixation, the syndesmosis can be tested. (*C*) A positive hook test shows syndesmotic insufficiency. Source: authors' drawing.

test. The hook test is used mainly to test syndesmotic stability, but, when lateralization of the talus is seen, this is proof of a deltoid ligament rupture (**Figs. 1** and **2**). The role of arthroscopy in detecting medial ligamentous injuries has been well investigated.[9,14,19]

TREATMENT

Many (narrative) reviews on whether to suture the deltoid ligament or not have been performed. There is a lack of high-quality studies with suturing the deltoid being the primary question. In 1987, Baird and Jackson[20] performed a review of the literature

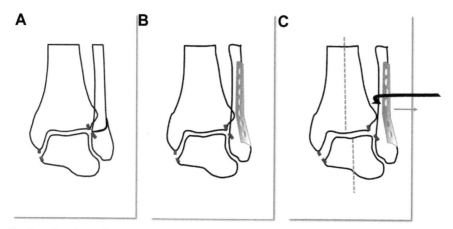

Fig. 2. When lateralization of the talus is seen, this is proof of a deltoid ligament rupture. (*A*) A typical trimalleolar fracture with a deltoid ligament rupture and a Weber B–type fibula fracture. (*B*) After plate fixation of the fibula, the interosseous membrane/ligament stabilizes the mortise, but usually not sufficiently. (*C*) A positive hook test shows syndesmotic and deltoid insufficiency. Source: authors' drawing.

on this topic. They found 12 articles that advocated surgical repair of the ligament and 9 studies that reported adequate results without surgical repair. However, the primary objective of these studies was not to evaluate the need for deltoid reconstruction, and the outcomes reported were to current standards rather than being descriptive and surgeon centered.[20] More recent reviews do show a trend toward concluding that there is an indication to suture the deltoid ligament, but up to the choice of the surgeon in which selected cases this is necessary.[21] One recent meta-analysis including 3 studies concluded that deltoid ligament repair in ankle fractures with a widened MCS showed a better anatomic reduction of the ankle, lower pain scores at final follow-up, and no significant increase in complication rate.[22]

Studies in Favor of Not Suturing the Deltoid Ligament

The authors found 4 comparative studies, with the need for suturing of the deltoid ligament as the primary question, that found it not necessary to explore and to reconstruct the deltoid ligament (**Table 1**).[20,23–25] The general consensus was that only if there is interposition on the medial side after adequate reduction in the fibular fracture is an exploration of the MCS required. Furthermore, there are several noncomparative studies specifically addressing the topic. Harper[26] treated 36 bimalleolar ankle fractures with the deltoid ligament equivalent without suturing the medial injury. The conclusion was that the deltoid ligament heals sufficiently with nonoperative treatment. Likewise, Zeegers and van der Werken[27] followed 28 patients with deltoid ruptures in ankle fractures for 18 months. All were not sutured. They concluded that, after anatomic reconstruction of the lateral malleolus with perfect congruity of the ankle mortise, there is no need to explore and suture the ruptured deltoid ligament. Another well-cited report is from Tourne and colleagues.[28] They treated 33 patients with fractures and followed them for 27 months, concluding to leave the ligament tears unexplored (medial, tibiofibular, and syndesmotic). As a result of these earlier studies, the current standard of practice in many centers is to restore the mortise anatomically and leave the deltoid complex to heal without direct surgical intervention.

Table 1				
Studies in favor of not suturing the deltoid ligament				
Study, Year	Patients (N)	Mean Follow-up (mo)	Sutured (N)	Conclusion
Baird & Jackson,[20] 1987	24	36	3	90% of the nonrepaired ligaments had a good or excellent result
Strömsöe et al,[23] 1995	50	17	25	A ruptured deltoid can be left unexplored. Operating time is reduced and the skin over the medial malleolus is left untouched
Maynou et al,[24] 1997	44	56	18	Repair of the deltoid ligament is unnecessary if the internal fixation of the fibula achieves an anatomic reconstruction of the mortise
Sun et al,[25] 2018	41	36	28	In conclusion, the results of this study do not support routine exposure and repairing of the injured deltoid ligaments

Studies in Favor of Suturing the Deltoid Ligament

The authors found 4 comparative studies with the need for suturing of the deltoid ligament as the primary question that found it necessary to explore and to reconstruct the deltoid ligament (**Table 2**).[29–32] The general consensus was that deltoid repair is able to restore congruity to the ankle joint, avoids the need to remove symptomatic syndesmotic implants, and is able to better reduce the MCS than syndesmotic implants. Furthermore, several noncomparative studies show that the deltoid ligament suture procedure is safe and effective.[33–35]

SURGICAL TECHNIQUE

Although several specific surgical techniques are used regarding deltoid ligament reconstruction in ankle fractures,[22,29,30,32–34,36–38] the general technique is as follows: an incision over the medial malleolus is made and an anteromedial arthrotomy is performed. The talar dome and medial gutter are inspected as well as the superficial and deep deltoid branches. The quality of the deltoid remnants is judged. Reinsertion to the medial malleolus or talus is performed by suturing directly to the bone, with suture anchors or with tape/graft through bone tunnels. In some cases, the tip of the malleolus or talus is prepared with a rongeur to promote osseoligamentous integration. In general, the primary ligamentous repair is achieved by using an absorbable suture material. Differences in surgical techniques are mostly related to the use of suture anchors to reinforce the repaired ligament, either which implant is used or whether

Table 2
Studies in favor of suturing the deltoid ligament

Study, Year	Patients (N)	Mean Follow-up (mo)	Sutured (N)	Conclusion
Jones & Nunley,[29] 2015	8	50	3	Deltoid repair is able to restore congruity to the ankle joint, and avoids the need to remove symptomatic syndesmotic implants
Zhao et al,[30] 2017	74	54	20	Surgical repair of the deltoid ligament is helpful in decreasing the postoperative MCS and malreduction rate, especially for the AO/OTA type C ankle fractures
Woo et al,[31] 2018	78	17	41	Although the clinical outcomes were not significantly different between the 2 groups, a more favorable final follow-up MCS was obtained in the deltoid repair group
Wu et al,[32] 2018	51	23	22	Deltoid ligament repair with a suture anchor had good functional and radiologic outcomes comparable with those with syndesmotic screw fixation but has a lower malreduction rate

Abbreviation: AO/OTA, AO Foundation/Orthopaedic Trauma Association.

implants are used at all. The suture anchors are used according to the manufacture's guidelines. Fluoroscopy is almost always used to ensure proper positioning of anchors and of the talus in the mortise. Manual stress testing is often applied to confirm appropriate MCS. Postoperatively, it is common practice to immobilize the patient in a short-leg cast for 2 to 6 weeks followed by aggressive range-of-motion and strengthening exercises under physical therapist guidance.

COMPLICATIONS OF DELTOID REPAIR

Dabash and colleagues[37] performed a systematic review after deltoid ligament repair and found complication rates to be lower in the repair group versus the nonrepair group (P = .0225). Superficial infection, medial instability, medial suture intolerance, algodystrophy, degenerative arthritis, and reoperation because of syndesmotic screw malposition were seen in the repair group, adding up to a total complication rate of 6.6%.[37] Also, more ossification of deltoid ligament was seen in the repair group.[24] The (extensive) medial approach results in a higher risk of wound breakdown and possible sequential wound infection. In nonaugmented non–allograft-reinforced repairs, the quality of the remnants is essential, as is the suture technique. In addition, the postoperative rehabilitation protocol should be as functional as possible to avoid a stiff ankle; however it must also protect the reconstruction.

COMPLICATIONS OF NOT SUTURING THE DELTOID

Dabash and colleagues[37] found a complication rate of 15.3% in the nonrepair group. Superficial infection, medial instability, reoperation because of syndesmotic screw malposition, failure, and reoperation because of symptomatic malreduction were seen. Nonanatomic healing of the deltoid ligament is the main concern because it can lead to substantial ankle instability with forthcoming posttraumatic instability osteoarthritis. Zhao and colleagues[30] reported substantial complications in the nonrepair group, which were not seen in the repair group, and these were all related to malreduction, with some requiring reoperation. However, medial instability has also been shown to result after both repairing and not repairing the deltoid ligament.[37] As reported by several investigators, there should be awareness of the possibility of a deltoid rupture in combination with a medial fracture.[14,39] The superficial component of the deltoid ligament is thin and weaker than the deep part and is under tension during external rotation of the ankle when the foot is in plantar flexion. Therefore, fixation of small anterior fractures of the medial malleolus, to which only the superficial portion of the ligament attaches, may not be sufficient to restore medial stability.[4,40]

FUTURE DIRECTIONS

General principles of ankle fracture treatment are based on restoring the mortise congruity and stability, in an attempt to avoid future posttraumatic arthritis.[41] Historically, this is done by means of fracture fixation with or without ligamentous stabilization. If rendered stable, early range-of-motion exercises are commenced as soon as tolerated. If the bony fixation is not stable, surgery is followed by plaster immobilization. If the ligaments are not augmented or repaired strongly, the plaster immobilization indirectly and statically allows the ligaments to heal. Although the lateral column is important, restoring fibula length and position, the medial column is probably more essential because the deltoid ligament is the medial restraint holding the talus under the tibia firmly, allowing less than 1 mm of lateralization.[12] In spite of the clinical relevance of the MCS, there remains a lack of consensus as to whether the deltoid ligament should be reconstructed.

In athletes, an algorithm was proposed by McCollum and colleagues[42] focusing on rapid recovery. They proposed to treat grade I and II sprains nonoperatively, whereas unstable grade III injuries with associated lateral ligament injuries may benefit from early surgical repair.[42,43] Early surgical repair has been advocated in athletes to ensure a rapid return to activity; although these studies are small regarding power and low in level of evidence, their reports on the low number of complications is favorable for surgical reconstruction adepts.[42–44] Future work should focus on 2 elements: the quality of direct repair/nonrepair comparative studies must be strengthened by means of level I randomized trials. Second, because research and development on anchors has improved over the years, these must be evaluated by means of rigorous clinical trials. Based on the currently available evidence, it is impossible to state whether there is a superior technique.

In cadaveric models of ankle fractures with deltoid ligament and/or syndesmotic disruption, joint contact forces remained abnormal even after anatomic reduction of the syndesmosis. Deltoid ligament repair after fibular fixation restored the position and stability of the talus in all planes of motion compared with the intact state. This outcome was not achieved with fibular fixation alone.[38,45] Earll and colleagues[46] showed that joint contact areas were decreased by 43% and peak cartilage pressures were increased by 30% after sectioning of the deltoid ligament. These findings support the clinical notion that a deltoid ligament rupture has to be put in a cast to heal, whereas a sutured deltoid ligament could render the ankle stable to perform early range-of-motion exercises.

The deltoid ligament has a close relationship with the syndesmotic ligaments.[47] When the syndesmosis is injured in isolation, an intact deltoid ligament restrains lateral talar displacement, and thereby tibiofibular diastasis, by indirectly tethering the distal fibula through the talus. In turn, when the deltoid ligament is additionally disrupted, this restraint is lost, generating the opportunity for syndesmotic instability. In cases where the syndesmotic stabilization is insufficient, the combination of deltoid ligament and syndesmotic rupture is a recipe for failure (**Fig. 3**). In these cases, additional deltoid ligament repair could strengthen the construct and stabilize the mortise. The study

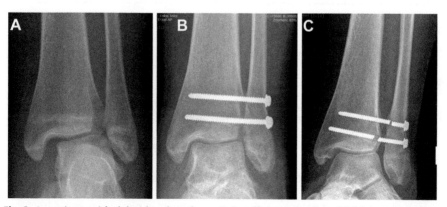

Fig. 3. In patients with deltoid and syndesmotic insufficiency (such as this Maisonneuve fracture seen in image *A*), syndesmotic stabilization alone (*B*) might not be sufficient (screw failure and lateralization of the talus as seen in *C*). A deltoid ligament repair can enhance the construct in these cases.

by Woo and colleagues[31] supports this clinically: a post hoc subgroup analysis was conducted in which only patients who also had syndesmotic injury were included. In this subgroup analysis, clinical outcomes were all superior in the deltoid repair group. These results suggest that deltoid repair may be clinically beneficial in patients who not only have deltoid rupture but also have syndesmotic injury.[31] The 2 repairs may reinforce each other and facilitate healing, especially in high fibula fractures (such as Maisonneuve fractures).

SUMMARY

The current literature supports both repair of the deltoid ligament and not repairing the deltoid in ankle fracture treatment. Exploration and reconstruction of the deltoid ligament are necessary if there is interposition on the medial side after adequate reduction of the fibular fracture. There may be an additional advantage of adding deltoid ligament repair for patients with obvious deltoid and syndesmotic injury. There also may be selected cases in which the deltoid ligament repair adds to the strength of the construct. Repositioning of the talus under the tibia (normalization of the MCS) is mandatory for a good outcome. In cases of doubt, arthroscopy could be of assistance to determine interposition when the MCS remains wide after proper reduction. There is no evidence proving superiority of suturing the deltoid ligament in all ruptures.

CLINICS CARE POINTS

- Diagnosing deltoid and syndesmotic ligament ruptures as part of ankle fractures is of paramount importance.
- The current literature supports both repair of the deltoid ligament and not repairing the deltoid in ankle fracture treatment.
- In small anterior colliculus fractures, be aware of concomitant deep deltoid ligament ruptures. Fixation of the small fragment alone does not provide medial stability.
- Exploration and reconstruction of the deltoid ligament are necessary if there is interposition on the medial side.
- There may be an additional advantage of adding deltoid ligament repair for patients with obvious deltoid and syndesmotic insufficiency.

DISCLOSURE

The authors have nothing to disclose.

REFERENCES

1. Michelson JD, Magid D, McHale K. Clinical utility of a stability-based ankle fracture classification system. J Orthop Trauma 2007;21(5):307–15.
2. Boden SD, Labropoulos PA, McCowin P, et al. Mechanical considerations for the syndesmosis screw. A cadaver study. J Bone Joint Surg Am 1989;71(10): 1548–55.
3. White TO. In defence of the posterior malleolus. Bone Joint J 2018;100-B(5): 566–9.
4. Tornetta P 3rd. Competence of the deltoid ligament in bimalleolar ankle fractures after medial malleolar fixation. J Bone Joint Surg Am 2000;82(6):843–8.
5. Somford MP, Wiegerinck JI, Hoornenborg D, et al. Ankle fracture eponyms. J Bone Joint Surg Am 2013;95(24). e198(1-7).

6. Lauge-Hansen N. Fractures of the ankle. II. Combined experimental-surgical and experimental-roentgenologic investigations. Arch Surg 1950;60(5):957–85.

7. Yde J, Kristensen KD. Ankle fractures: supination-eversion fractures of stage IV. Primary and late results of operative and non-operative treatment. Acta Orthop Scand 1980;51(6):981–90.

8. Donken CC, van Laarhoven CJ, Edwards MJ, et al. Misdiagnosis of OTA type B (Weber B) ankle fractures leading to nonunion. J Foot Ankle Surg 2011;50(4): 430–3.

9. Hintermann B, Regazzoni P, Lampert C, et al. Arthroscopic findings in acute fractures of the ankle. J Bone Joint Surg Br 2000;82(3):345–51.

10. Lindsjo U. Operative treatment of ankle fracture-dislocations. A follow-up study of 306/321 consecutive cases. Clin Orthop Relat Res 1985;199:28–38.

11. Jehlicka D, Bartonicek J, Svatos F, et al. [Fracture-dislocations of the ankle joint in adults. Part I: epidemiologic evaluation of patients during a 1-year period]. Acta Chir Orthop Traumatol Cech 2002;69(4):243–7.

12. Rasmussen O, Kromann-Andersen C, Boe S. Deltoid ligament. Functional analysis of the medial collateral ligamentous apparatus of the ankle joint. Acta Orthop Scand 1983;54(1):36–44.

13. DeAngelis NA, Eskander MS, French BG. Does medial tenderness predict deep deltoid ligament incompetence in supination-external rotation type ankle fractures? J Orthop Trauma 2007;21(4):244–7.

14. Schuberth JM, Collman DR, Rush SM, et al. Deltoid ligament integrity in lateral malleolar fractures: a comparative analysis of arthroscopic and radiographic assessments. J Foot Ankle Surg 2004;43(1):20–9.

15. Henari S, Banks LN, Radovanovic I, et al. Ultrasonography as a diagnostic tool in assessing deltoid ligament injury in supination external rotation fractures of the ankle. Orthopedics 2011;34(10):e639–43.

16. Chen PY, Wang TG, Wang CL. Ultrasonographic examination of the deltoid ligament in bimalleolar equivalent fractures. Foot Ankle Int 2008;29(9):883–6.

17. Crim J, Longenecker LG. MRI and surgical findings in deltoid ligament tears. AJR Am J Roentgenol 2015;204(1):W63–9.

18. Gardner MJ, Demetrakopoulos D, Briggs SM, et al. The ability of the Lauge-Hansen classification to predict ligament injury and mechanism in ankle fractures: an MRI study. J Orthop Trauma 2006;20(4):267–72.

19. Chun KY, Choi YS, Lee SH, et al. Deltoid ligament and tibiofibular syndesmosis injury in chronic lateral ankle instability: magnetic resonance imaging evaluation at 3T and comparison with arthroscopy. Korean J Radiol 2015;16(5):1096–103.

20. Baird RA, Jackson ST. Fractures of the distal part of the fibula with associated disruption of the deltoid ligament. Treatment without repair of the deltoid ligament. J Bone Joint Surg Am 1987;69(9):1346–52.

21. Lee S, Lin J, Hamid KS, et al. Deltoid ligament rupture in ankle fracture: diagnosis and management. J Am Acad Orthop Surg 2019;27(14):e648–58.

22. Salameh M, Alhammoud A, Alkhatib N, et al. Outcome of primary deltoid ligament repair in acute ankle fractures: a meta-analysis of comparative studies. Int Orthop 2020;44(2):341–7.

23. Stromsoe K, Hoqevold HE, Skjeldal S, et al. The repair of a ruptured deltoid ligament is not necessary in ankle fractures. J Bone Joint Surg Br 1995;77(6):920–1.

24. Maynou C, Lesage P, Mestdagh H, et al. [Is surgical treatment of deltoid ligament rupture necessary in ankle fractures?]. Rev Chir Orthop Reparatrice Appar Mot 1997;83(7):652–7.

25. Sun X, Li T, Sun Z, et al. Does routinely repairing deltoid ligament injuries in type B ankle joint fractures influence long term outcomes? Injury 2018;49(12):2312–7.

26. Harper MC. The deltoid ligament. An evaluation of need for surgical repair. Clin Orthop Relat Res 1988;(226):156–68.

27. Zeegers AV, van der Werken C. Rupture of the deltoid ligament in ankle fractures: should it be repaired? Injury 1989;20(1):39–41.

28. Tourne Y, Charbel A, Picard F, et al. Surgical treatment of bi- and trimalleolar ankle fractures: should the medial collateral ligament be sutured or not? J Foot Ankle Surg 1999;38(1):24–9.

29. Jones CR, Nunley JA 2nd. Deltoid ligament repair versus syndesmotic fixation in bimalleolar equivalent ankle fractures. J Orthop Trauma 2015;29(5):245–9.

30. Zhao HM, Lu J, Zhang F, et al. Surgical treatment of ankle fracture with or without deltoid ligament repair: a comparative study. BMC Musculoskelet Disord 2017; 18(1):543.

31. Woo SH, Bae SY, Chung HJ. Short-term results of a ruptured deltoid ligament repair during an acute ankle fracture fixation. Foot Ankle Int 2018;39(1):35–45.

32. Wu K, Lin J, Huang J, et al. Evaluation of transsyndesmotic fixation and primary deltoid ligament repair in ankle fractures with suspected combined deltoid ligament injury. J Foot Ankle Surg 2018;57(4):694–700.

33. Yu GR, Zhang MZ, Aiyer A, et al. Repair of the acute deltoid ligament complex rupture associated with ankle fractures: a multicenter clinical study. J Foot Ankle Surg 2015;54(2):198–202.

34. Hardy MA, Connors JC, Zulauf EE, et al. Acute deltoid ligament repair in ankle fractures: five-year follow-up. Clin Podiatr Med Surg 2020;37(2):295–304.

35. Johnson DP, Hill J. Fracture-dislocation of the ankle with rupture of the deltoid ligament. Injury 1988;19(2):59–61.

36. Rigby RB, Scott RT. Role for primary repair of deltoid ligament complex in ankle fractures. Clin Podiatr Med Surg 2018;35(2):183–97.

37. Dabash S, Elabd A, Potter E, et al. Adding deltoid ligament repair in ankle fracture treatment: Is it necessary? A systematic review. Foot Ankle Surg 2019;25(6): 714–20.

38. Butler BA, Hempen EC, Barbosa M, et al. Deltoid ligament repair reduces and stabilizes the talus in unstable ankle fractures. J Orthop 2020;17:87–90.

39. Pai VS. Medial malleolar fracture associated with deltoid ligament rupture. J Foot Ankle Surg 1999;38(6):420–2.

40. Stufkens SA, van den Bekerom MP, Knupp M, et al. The diagnosis and treatment of deltoid ligament lesions in supination-external rotation ankle fractures: a review. Strateg Trauma Limb Reconstr 2012;7(2):73–85.

41. Stufkens SA, van den Bekerom MP, Kerkhoffs GM, et al. Long-term outcome after 1822 operatively treated ankle fractures: a systematic review of the literature. Injury 2011;42(2):119–27.

42. McCollum GA, van den Bekerom MP, Kerkhoffs GM, et al. Syndesmosis and deltoid ligament injuries in the athlete. Knee Surg Sports Traumatol Arthrosc 2013; 21(6):1328–37.

43. Calder JD, Bamford R, Petrie A, et al. Stable Versus Unstable Grade II high ankle sprains: a prospective study predicting the need for surgical stabilization and time to return to sports. Arthroscopy 2016;32(4):634–42.

44. Hsu AR, Lareau CR, Anderson RB. Repair of acute superficial deltoid complex avulsion during ankle fracture fixation in national football league players. Foot Ankle Int 2015;36(11):1272–8.

45. LaMothe J, Baxter JR, Gilbert S, et al. Effect of complete syndesmotic disruption and deltoid injuries and different reduction methods on ankle joint contact mechanics. Foot Ankle Int 2017;38(6):694–700.

46. Earll M, Wayne J, Brodrick C, et al. Contribution of the deltoid ligament to ankle joint contact characteristics: a cadaver study. Foot Ankle Int 1996;17(6):317–24.

47. Massri-Pugin J, Lubberts B, Vopat BG, et al. Role of the deltoid ligament in syndesmotic instability. Foot Ankle Int 2018;39(5):598–603.

Current Concepts in Treatment of Ligament Incompetence in the Acquired Flatfoot

Emilio Wagner, MD*, Pablo Wagner, MD

KEYWORDS

- Ligament insufficiency • Flatfoot • Deltoid ligament • Spring ligament
- Tibiocalcaneonavicular ligament • Flatfoot algorithm

KEY POINTS

- Flatfoot is a complex deformity with multiligamentous insufficiency.
- Skeletal and soft tissue reconstruction must be considered when considering operative intervention.
- Ankle, hindfoot, and midfoot must be considered in the analysis when planning a flatfoot reconstruction.
- Tibiocalcaneonavicular ligament reconstruction should be considered in almost every flexible flatfoot case.

INTRODUCTION

Adult-acquired flatfoot consists of a flattened foot, with a combination of deformities, such as a flat arch, valgus hindfoot, and varying degrees of forefoot abduction. The deformity can vary in severity and location and often results in a progressive deterioration of foot function. Historically considered because of a posterior tibial tendon failure, a combination of ligament insufficiencies has been shown to be present, which explains the multiple apices of deformity generally present in flatfeet cases.[1] The multiple sites of deformity explain the wide variation on its clinical presentation.[2] Pain initially may be present along the medial aspect of the ankle joint, or in relation to the posterior tibial tendon, which becomes inflamed because of its continued pull of trying to hold the hindfoot and medial arch. Later in its natural history, flatfoot pain may propagate along the medial arch itself and even progress onto the lateral aspect of the ankle because of subfibular impingement. In this article, the authors analyze the

Universidad del Desarrollo, Clinica Alemana de Santiago, Vitacura 5951, Santiago, Chile
* Corresponding author.
E-mail address: ewagner@alemana.cl

Foot Ankle Clin N Am 26 (2021) 373–389
https://doi.org/10.1016/j.fcl.2021.03.010
1083-7515/21/© 2021 Elsevier Inc. All rights reserved.

current concepts in treatment of ligament incompetence of the acquired flatfoot, considering the skeletal actions recommended to achieve deformity correction and the soft tissue reconstructions to repair or strengthen the damaged ligaments. The flatfeet history, study, and diagnostic aspects are out of the scope of this article.

BIOMECHANICAL BACKGROUND

One of the first manifestations of flatfoot deformity is a decrease in the medial longitudinal arch.[3] To observe a loss in medial arch height, the main tissues capable of supporting the arch must become involved, that is, the plantar fascia, the spring ligament, and the tibialis posterior tendon.[4] Furthermore, in this last study, it was also shown that the posterior tibial tendon itself is not able to support the plantar arch itself, which supports the concept of a multiple ligament deficiency pathologic condition. Besides statically becoming a flatfoot, kinematic alterations, such as calcaneal eversion, internal tibial rotation, and abduction of the forefoot, will occur.[5] Hindfoot eversion will further increase the chance of deformity progression, as the Achilles tendon becomes a deforming vector/force. Once talocalcaneal rotation happens, more stress will be translated onto medial structures, such as the deltoid, spring ligament, and the talonavicular joint.[6] A recent study showed that there is a strong connection between the navicular and medial cuneiform, which highlights the multiple ligament connection between the medial column and the hindfoot.[7] The windlass mechanism produced by the plantar fascia dynamically stabilizes the medial column through its attachment to the calcaneus and forefoot (ie, sesamoid bones, plantar plates of lesser metatarsals, plantar fat pad). In the propulsive phase of gait, the windlass mechanism shortens the plantar aponeurosis, which helps to create a rigid medial column, necessary for toe-off.[8] For this important function to happen, the windlass mechanism relies on healthy functioning joints and ligaments. Therefore, any incompetence of the medial column joints may result in a deficiency of this mechanism and loss of function and improper gait mechanics.

Multiple classifications have been proposed to provide guidelines in the analysis and treatment of acquired flatfeet.[9] They are mainly based on foot position and deformity flexibility. Radiographic analysis considers axial weight-bearing radiographs, which provide alignment views useful to measure the distance between the mechanical axis of the tibia and the point of contact between the calcaneus and the floor.[10] Foot anteroposterior (AP) and lateral weight-bearing views provide useful information relative to the talocalcaneal rotation, talonavicular relation, and any medial column sag or instability present. The authors prefer to analyze flatfeet deformities from a biomechanical perspective, from proximal to distal, considering the location of the apex of the deformity, and thus propose treatment depending on where the apices are, and how severe the deformity is. Ligament reconstruction is considered whenever the deformity is flexible, with or without arthritis. Flexible deformities are defined by the authors as any clinical malalignment that can be corrected actively by the patient, or passively by the physician (considering intraoperative manipulation, usually controlled by fluoroscopy). In this way, the proposed algorithm for analysis for reconstructive procedures in flexible flatfoot is presented in **Fig. 1**.

FLEXIBLE FLATFOOT INSTABILITY ANALYSIS
Supramalleolar Apex

The analysis starts at the supramalleolar region, where the coronal and sagittal plane alignment must be analyzed in search of any deformity, being normal values of the distal anterolateral angle of the tibia between 88° and 95° and the anterior distal angle

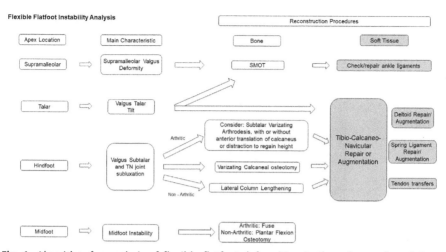

Fig. 1. Algorithm for analysis of flexible flatfeet deformities. In the columns from left to right are the apex location of the deformity, the main radiological characteristic, the bone reconstruction procedures, and the soft tissue reconstruction procedures (*gray shading*). SMOT, supramalleolar osteotomy; TN, talonavicular joint.

of the tibia between 78° and 82°.[11,12] Corrective supramalleolar or even intraarticular osteotomies can be planned when any malalignment is found in this region (**Fig. 2**).

Talar Apex

The talus should be evaluated in its mortise, and no tilt should be found in relation to the pilon. The talar tilt angle can be measured as the difference between the distal lateral angle of the tibia and the tibiotalar angle, measured between the mechanical axis of the tibia and the most superior surface of the talus. The normal value is 0° to 4°. If altered, it means either there is an asymmetric wear of the cartilage, that is, a localized arthrosis of the ankle joint,[13] or there is a medial deltoid ligament instability of the ankle joint.[2] When correcting a talar tilt, after corrective osteotomies or arthrodesis is made, if the talus maintains a tilted situation inside the ankle joint and imaging studies confirm isolated damage of the deltoid ligament, a reconstruction of the deltoid complex should be considered.

Hindfoot Apex

Whenever there is a loss of height at the hindfoot, the talus may rotate or tilt because of the loss of intrinsic stability, showing signs of peritalar instability.[14] Instability may manifest in diverse forms, such as coronal deviation in varus or valgus, sagittal deformities, such as plantar flexion or dorsiflexion, and finally, axial deviation, such as internal or external rotation.[15] The reader is referred to Beat Hintermann and Roxa Ruiz's article "Biomechanics of Medial Ankle and Peritalar Instability" and Yantarat Sripanich and Alexej Barg's article "Imaging of Peritalar Instability" in this issue to learn more about this topic. More distally, the subtalar joint can compensate 58% and 35% of the varus and valgus deviation, respectively, at the ankle joint.[16] Deformity at the subtalar joint is fundamental to evaluate, as it may be part of a peritalar instability or already be one of the components of a rigid flatfoot deformity. One way to measure subtalar malalignment uses the hindfoot alignment angle. This angle is defined by the intersection between the tibial and calcaneal axis[17] (**Fig. 3**). Hindfoot malalignment represents a coronal rotation

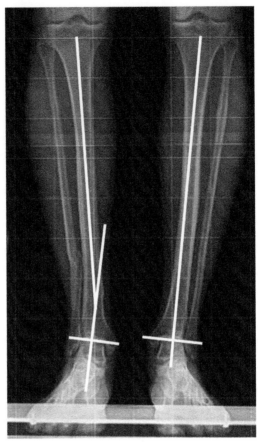

Fig. 2. Full-length leg radiograph of patient where, on the left side, a clear valgus orientation of the distal tibia is observed, generating a supramalleolar valgus deformity.

of the talus over the calcaneus, specifically, an external rotation of the calcaneus in relation to the talus.[3] As the tibia internally rotates and the calcaneus everts, more pressure is translated onto the talonavicular joint, and an abduction deformity of the forefoot over the hindfoot may occur.[6] If the flatfoot deformity increases, at this point, a more severe ligament insufficiency of the medial ankle and midfoot is expected to be present. As the medial ligament insufficiency progresses, a multiplanar instability of the ankle develops, because of erosion and wear of the calcaneofibular ligament.[13] Because of this, a combined ligament repair should be performed in these cases. A recent anatomic study analyzed the medial ankle ligament complex as a functional unit and defined the largest component of the deltoid as the tibiocalcaneonavicular ligament, which apparently includes portions of the tibionavicular, tibiospring, and tibiocalcaneal ligaments.[18] In summary, whenever the talus is malrotated over the calcaneus, after corrective osteotomies or arthrodesis are made, a tibiocalcaneonavicular reconstruction and a lateral ligament repair or reconstruction may be considered.

Midfoot Apex

Medial column stability is crucial to evaluate in flatfoot patients. On lateral weight-bearing radiographs, any loss of the medial longitudinal arch must be measured,

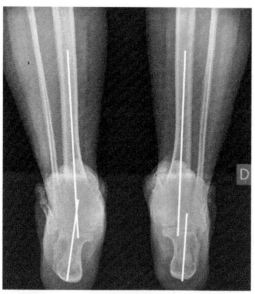

Fig. 3. Bilateral axial hindfoot radiograph showing the hindfoot alignment angle, between the tibia axis and the calcaneal axis. In this example, a clear increase in deformity is seen on the left side of the picture.

that is, any loss in height between the lateral and the medial column. Any collapse seen on radiographs indicates insufficiency of the pertaining ligaments of that joint **(Fig. 4)**. Collapse can occur through the talonavicular, naviculocuneiform, cuneome-tatarsal, or combination of these joints.[9] The most named ligament in this area is the spring ligament, frequently damaged in flatfeet, and even isolated tears of it can produce a flatfoot condition.[19] This condition constitutes what has been named a forefoot-driven hindfoot valgus deformity, where no real pathologic condition is found in the hindfoot, which may explain the pathologic valgus, but instead a pathologic medial column is present, allowing the midfoot and forefoot to lose height, thereby pulling the hindfoot into valgus. A medial column insufficiency with a sag at the talonavicular or naviculocuneiform joint, after corrective osteotomies or arthrodesis, may be amenable for reconstruction with spring ligament repairs or naviculocuneiform repairs.

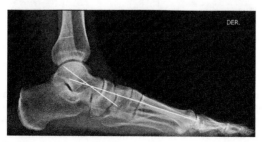

Fig. 4. Lateral weight-bearing foot radiograph of a symptomatic flatfoot patient. Notice the abnormal Meary angle drawn between the axis of the talus and the first metatarsal bone. No clear sag is seen in any specific joint, but rather a diffuse loss of Meary angle.

FLEXIBLE FLATFOOT INSTABILITY TREATMENT

No published algorithm evaluates the apex of deformity in a flatfoot condition in a proximal-to-distal manner. The authors think that a proximal-to-distal analysis helps to organize better the treatment alternatives, from a skeletal and soft tissue point of view. Depending on the level of the deformity, different reconstruction procedures can be applied, dividing them into bone procedures or soft tissue procedures (see **Fig. 1**). The authors briefly analyze the different treatment alternatives depending on the apex of the deformity location, first naming the skeletal procedures and then the soft tissue repair or reconstruction. In this issue, separate articles include deltoid and spring ligament repair (See Gastón Slullitel and Juan Pablo Calvi's article "Current Concepts in Treatment of Acute Deltoid Instability", Cesar de Cesar Netto and John E. Femino's article "State of the Art in Treatment of Chronic Medial Ankle Instability" and Caio Nery and Daniel Baumfeld's article "Current Trends in Treatment of Injuries to Spring Ligament"). Therefore, in this article, the authors focus on hindfoot correction through a combined deltoid and spring ligament approach, which they name as the tibiocalcaneonavicular ligament repair and reconstruction.

Supramalleolar Valgus Deformity

Bone reconstruction

A supramalleolar osteotomy (SMOT) is well suited to address almost any kind of supramalleolar deformity and intraarticular deformities, even where asymmetric

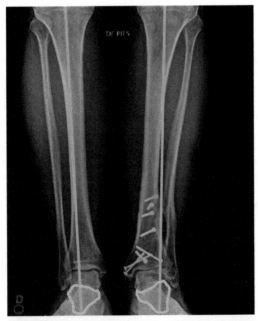

Fig. 5. AP weight-bearing leg radiographs, in which an old distal tibia fracture can be noted on the left leg (*right side of the image*). Note the intraarticular valgus alignment of the talus, owing to an asymmetric posttraumatic ankle arthrosis where more damage was sustained on the lateral aspect of the joint. The mechanical axes are drawn on each leg for comparison (*blue lines*), and the calcaneus silhouettes are depicted as orange lines. Note the lateralization of the weight-bearing axis of the left leg, where the blue line crosses the ankle joint at the level of the tibiofibular joint.

arthrosis is present. An example of a supramalleolar valgus deformity is presented in **Fig. 2**. In cases of asymmetric arthrosis of the ankle joint, more cartilage loss can be found in the lateral aspect of the ankle joint, on either the talar or the tibial side, producing an intraarticular valgus deformity (**Fig. 5**). In these supramaleolar deformities, a medial closing wedge SMOT is generally recommended, with a medial tibial wedge resection considering the whole foot for final balance[13] (**Fig. 6**).

Soft tissue reconstruction

As commented previously in the instability analysis section, these patients frequently develop a multiplanar instability of the ankle. Because of this, a combined ligament repair should be performed. The medial ligaments must be examined, as continuous stress may have deteriorated their insertion. Relevant to this damage is to correctly identify the insufficient components, and most frequently the tibionavicular and tibiospring components are compromised.[20] In these cases, reattachment with bony anchors placed at the navicular and at the distal tibia is recommended. The lateral ligaments must be tested under fluoroscopy, and if lax, their insufficiency should also be addressed at the same time of the osteotomy.

Valgus Talar Tilt

Bone reconstruction

Almost every talar tilt presents some amount of asymmetric ankle cartilage damage, which allows the talus to tilt inside the mortise. Whenever the talus is tilted into valgus inside the mortise, a peritalar instability should be suspected. Peritalar instability has been analyzed by Hintermann and colleagues[13,14] and is analyzed elsewhere in this issue. If there is arthrosis present at the peritalar joints, regaining stability through

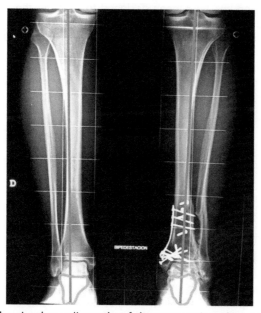

Fig. 6. AP weight-bearing leg radiographs of the same patient shown in **Fig. 5**. A medial closing wedge SMOT was performed on the left leg (*right side of the image*) achieving a medialization of the weight-bearing axis (note where the *blue line* crosses the ankle joint). The calcaneal silhouette is marked with an orange line. A good clinical result was achieved and lasted for 10 years.

subtalar arthrodesis, triple arthrodesis, or subtalar distraction arthrodesis is a definitive solution that will regain hindfoot height and through that regain tension of the ligaments and soft tissues, improving ankle stability.[21–23] Final alignment is achieved adding a medial closing wedge SMOT (**Figs. 7** and **8**). If no arthrosis is present at the peritalar joints, valgus talar tilt can be managed solely through a medial closing wedge SMOT. In these selected cases, after performing the SMOT, intraoperative fluoroscopy is mandatory to evaluate the correct realignment of the talus inside the mortise, adding soft tissue reconstructions as needed.

Soft tissue reconstruction

It must be remembered that isolated deltoid ligament damage is seldom present, and the authors recommend almost always performing combined tibiocalcaneonavicular repairs or reconstruction (see next section). For isolated deltoid ligament damage, the authors refer the reader to review the topic in this issue (see Jordi Vega and Matteo Guelfi's article "Arthroscopic Assessment and Treatment of Medial Collateral Ligament Complex", Gastón Slullitel and Juan Pablo Calvi's article "Current Concepts in Treatment of Acute Deltoid Instability" and Cesar de Cesar Netto and John E. Femino's article "State of the Art in Treatment of Chronic Medial Ankle Instability").

Subtalar Valgus and Talonavicular Joint Deformity

Bone reconstruction

For a subtalar joint valgus deformity to appear, it has been already mentioned that a talocalcaneal rotation must occur, which includes an internal rotation of the talus with a secondary talonavicular incongruency and valgus deformity of the hindfoot. Different bony procedures have been designed to derotate the talus in relation to the calcaneus and decrease medial soft tissue strain, namely subtalar arthrodesis, and varus producing calcaneal and lateral column lengthening osteotomies. When

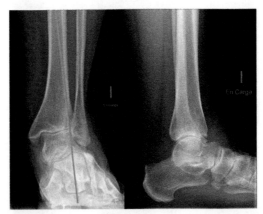

Fig. 7. AP weight-bearing ankle radiograph of a severe flatfoot case with valgus ankle, valgus hindfoot, and peritalar instability. The blue line represents the mechanical axis of the limb, which crosses the ankle join at the tibiofibular joint. The calcaneus silhouette is represented with an orange line. See the lateral ankle view, where a subluxation of the talonavicular and subtalar joint can be seen. In this case, a triple arthrodesis could align the hindfoot but would not correct the valgus ankle. To realign the mechanical axis, an SMOT must be added.

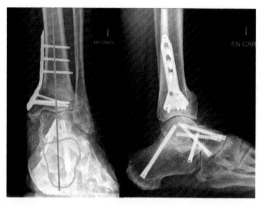

Fig. 8. AP weight-bearing ankle radiographs of the same patient shown in **Fig. 7**. The blue line now intersects the ankle joint line in the middle of the joint. The calcaneal silhouette is marked with an orange line. The stability and height of the hindfoot were restored thanks to the arthrodesis. Note that although a medial closing wedge SMOT was added, the ankle joint line still remains in a slight valgus. This exemplifies how important it was to add an SMOT in this case, as a triple arthrodesis alone would have been completely insufficient. It also shows the difficulty in achieving excellent alignments in these cases.

there is already a symptomatic arthritis at the subtalar joint, a subtalar corrective arthrodesis is the treatment of choice, which will correct rotation, eversion, and valgus malalignment of the calcaneus in relation to the talus.

A subtalar corrective arthrodesis must correct all the components of the deformity, including the external rotation of the calcaneus in relation to the talus, the consequent valgus of the subtalar joint, and the loss of hindfoot height. The apex of the hindfoot deformity in a flatfoot case lies on the posterior facet of the subtalar joint, which corresponds to the center of rotation of the subtalar joint. In relation to this apex, the talus rotates on top of the calcaneus, falling into valgus, losing height, and creating a midfoot deformity. A corrective arthrodesis therefore should be performed, producing an

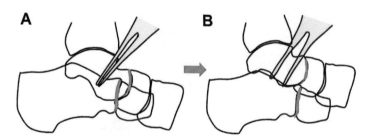

Fig. 9. (A) A flatfoot hindfoot, from the lateral view. The maneuver to derotate the talus in relation to the calcaneus uses a lamina spreader, drawn in the image as a yellow figure. The arms of the spreader are placed against the floor of the sinus tarsi distally and plantarly, and against the anterolateral process of the talus, proximally and dorsally. (B) The lamina spreader is shown opened, and the derotation of the talus on the calcaneus is evident. Now the talus sits on top of the calcaneus, and because of the distraction, the calcaneus is brought forward in relation to the talus, thus creating a lateral column lengthening effect. Note the chopart joint, depicted as a blue area, as it changes from A to B, becoming well aligned in panel B.

internal rotation of the calcaneus in relation to the talus. Achieving this derotation corrects the hindfoot height and valgus, as the talus recovers its original position, and may improve ankle stability because of medial deltoid ligament retensioning. The authors recommend, when performing a subtalar arthrodesis, to focus intraoperatively in derotating the talus on the calcaneus. This maneuver is performed using a lamina spreader placed against the floor of the sinus tarsi and against the anterolateral process of the talus (**Fig. 9**). A distraction between the 2 points pushes the talus backwards and rotates it externally, achieving a derotation and also a relative lengthening of the lateral column, which also assists in correcting any abduction deformity at the talonavicular joint (**Fig. 10**).

If the subtalar joint is not arthritic, a medial translational calcaneal osteotomy may be of use. Caution must be taken if there is any concern about peritalar instability. In some cases, because of some cartilage loss at the ankle joint, a varizating calcaneal osteotomy may create a zigzag effect, which has been described where an increase in the valgus orientation of the hindfoot may occur.[24] Finally, the last skeletal option to correct a subtalar and talonavicular malalignment is a lateral column lengthening. This procedure can be performed through a classic anterior process, calcaneal osteotomy, or through a step cut osteotomy of the calcaneus.[25] The correction of the talocalcaneal rotational deformity through a lateral column lengthening occurs through the talonavicular joint, where the calcaneus pushes forward the lateral column, thereby correcting the abduction deformity and secondarily pushing the talus over the calcaneus in a corrected position. It has been shown that lengthening the calcaneus is highly effective to correct abduction,[26] and its correction capacity has been measured.[27] A limit between 4 and 8 mm of lengthening has been proposed[26] because of concerns of hindfoot rigidity, lateral column overload, and inferior functional outcomes observed after excessive lateral column lengthening. These concerns highlight the difficulty in achieving a deformity correction beneficial for the patient. It may be possible to avoid overcorrection through lateral column lengthening restricting its use, indicating it after

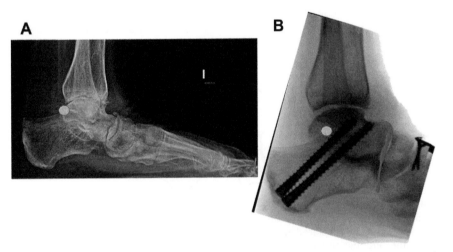

Fig. 10. (*A*) Intraoperative fluoroscopy depicting the same maneuver shown in **Fig. 9**. The chopart joint is delineated with blue lines. The yellow dot is sitting on the most posterior aspect of the calcaneus. (*B*) Note how after the derotation arthrodesis, the chopart joint now is well aligned and how the calcaneus now lies anteriorly displaced in relation to the talus.

certain deformity limit, for example, 50% of talonavicular uncoverage. For cases under this limit, a combined deltoid and spring soft tissue retensioning and reconstruction could be beneficial.[9,28] This last approach is the one the authors recommend, and it is detailed in the next section.

Soft tissue reconstruction

Tibiocalcaneonavicular reconstruction. A complex combination of soft tissue damage must be assumed to be present in these cases, that is, the calcaneonavicular (spring) ligament, posterior tibialis tendon, deltoid ligament, plantar fascia, short and long plantar ligament, joint capsules, and intrinsic foot muscles, among others. Of all these structures, the most important is the plantar fascia, which provides 25% of arch stiffness.[29] The reconstruction of the spring, deltoid, or any other ligament in isolation will probably not be enough to support the longitudinal arch and medial mid-rearfoot structures, given that medial ligaments work as a unit.[18] The proposed reconstruction should include every damaged medial structure and not just segments of it, following the concept of a tibiocalcaneonavicular reconstrucion. This reconstruction closely resembles the whole medial rearfoot ligament complex: tibiocalcaneal, tibiospring, tibionavicular, and calcaneonavicular ligaments (**Fig. 11**). There are some publications regarding this combined comprehensive reconstruction. In 2010, Williams and colleagues[30] compared different spring ligament reconstructions, namely, a calcaneonavicular and a deltoid-navicular configuration. The deltoid-navicular reconstruction was able to correct more degrees of midfoot abduction than the calcaneonavicular one. This cadaveric study was later supported by a finite element analysis in which a

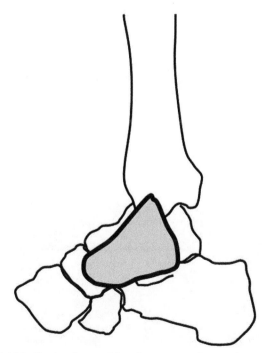

Fig. 11. The medial hindfoot, where a triangle was superimposed over the area between the tibia, calcaneus, and navicular. This triangle represents the tibiocalcaneonavicular ligament.

reconstruction from the medial cuneiform to the medial malleolus was the best option for controlling midfoot abduction.[31] In 2014, Baxter and colleagues[32] performed a study that showed that a tibionavicular reconstruction was better than a spring ligament reconstruction in restoring normal foot kinematics. To the best of the authors' knowledge, Grunfeld and colleagues[33] in 2016 were the first authors to report a surgical technique for the combined reconstruction of the deltoid and spring ligament. They described an allograft technique attached to the medial malleolus and using 2 limbs to have attachments at the sustentaculum tali and at the navicular. One year later, Patel and colleagues[28] described another combined reconstruction using synthetically augmented grafts on tibionavicular and tibiotalar directions, with good clinical results in a small series of patients. A reinforcement of native deltoid and spring ligaments with synthetic tape has also been published, that is, tibiotalar, tibiocalcaneal, and calcaneonavicular, with good initial results.[34] In 2019, Brodell and colleagues[35] analyzed Grunfeld's technique and added a modification that included a limb specifically for the spring ligament using tendon allograft. This modification has the advantage of reconstructing the whole medial ligament structures with an allograft, including the calcaneonavicular segment. This modification is the most complete medial ligament reconstruction published nowadays.

The authors' current recommendation is to perform a comprehensive reconstruction, including the tibionavicular, tibiocalcaneal, and calcaneonavicular ligaments for flexible flatfoot, in a similar fashion as Brodell has published. This reconstruction has a triangular shape that consolidates the hindfoot and midfoot medial soft tissue wall. Three tunnel points of fixation are recommended: one on the medial malleolus exiting laterally at the tibia for better fixation; one at the navicular tuberosity (tunnel in a plantar-dorsal direction); and one at the sustentaculum tali (exits laterally at the calcaneus). Whether tendon (auto or allograft) or synthetic augmentation is used, it depends on the native ligament's quality. When no ligament degeneration exists and insufficient but present ligaments are the case, an augmentation using suture-tape synthetic material is recommended (ultra-high-molecular-weight polyethylene, UHMWP) in addition to osseous procedures. If ligamentous degeneration exists, or no ligaments are present whatsoever, a reconstruction using a tendon allograft (peroneus longus, for example) or autograft (gracilis, semitendinosus) is recommended. For these reconstructions, a synthetic augmentation in addition to the tendon is the ideal construct. This combination of tendon graft and synthetic material avoids the tendon graft lengthening that inevitably occurs over time.

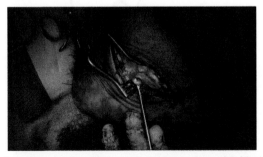

Fig. 12. Intraoperative picture of medial surgical approach to the hindfoot, between the medial malleolus and the navicular bone, identifying the flexor hallucis longus in order to locate the sustentaculum tali. *Courtesy of* Dr Anish R. Kadakia MD, Chicago, Illinois.

The surgical technique recommended by the authors (performed at the end of all osseous procedures) is described as follows:

The approach is from the medial malleolus tip to the naviculocuneiform joint. Expose and identify medial malleolus tip, tibialis posterior, and navicular tuberosity (**Fig. 12**). Identify ligaments sufficiency and tibialis posterior degeneration. If a tendon allograft will be used, measure its width to choose the appropriate drill bit. The recommended tendon width is 4 to 5 mm, and the minimum recommended length is 25 cm. Perform the medial malleolar tunnel, starting at the malleolar tip in 45° of superolateral direction, until the lateral tibial cortex is crossed. At the navicular tuberosity, drill from inferomedial to superomedial. At the sustentaculum tali, start drilling 5 mm below the articular surface in 15° of plantar inclination (to avoid subtalar joint penetration) until the lateral calcaneal cortex is breached. The tibial tunnel should be 3 mm bigger than the tendon width, given that a folded tendon will be inserted through these tunnels. Suture each tendon end in a Krackow fashion or using a suture loop. Keep the tendon under tension at a side table for 5 minutes.

Start by traversing 1 tendon end through the calcaneal tunnel and transiently secure the sutures laterally at the calcaneus with a clamp. Then, insert the other tendon end through the navicular tunnel from plantar to dorsal. At least 1 cm of each tendon end should fit inside the calcaneal and navicular tunnels. Leave the sutures exiting laterally at the calcaneus and dorsally at the navicular clamped for later tendon tensioning. Finally, fold and suture the tendon remnant on a suture loop attached to a suture button (anterior cruciate ligament button can be used). Insert this button through the tibial tunnel. Make a 2-cm approach laterally at the tibia for suture-button retrieval. Apply light tension to the tendon graft by pulling at the button sutures. Make sure both tendon ends are still in their respective tunnels. Secure this button by 3 double knots at the lateral tibia. Insert an interference screw at the tibial malleolus tunnel for double graft fixation. Proceed then by inserting 1 end of a suture-tape material (UHMWP) into the sustentaculum tali tunnel and the other into the navicular. The suture tape emulates the spring ligament. Now, use an interference screw at the navicular to fix the suture tape and tendon graft while applying tension to the tendon graft. Then, focus on the calcaneus tunnel. Apply tension to the suture tape and tendon end at their exit through the lateral calcaneus wall, while an assistant holds the foot in the neutral position. Use a button (at the lateral calcaneal wall) and an interference screw at the sustentaculum tali for double graft fixation. Finally, reinforce the whole tendon allograft with a nonresorbable suture (UHMWP material). This reinforcement will give a more rigid structure to the whole tendon graft, avoiding tendon lengthening (**Fig. 13**). In relation to tendon transfers, the authors do not recommend resecting the tibialis posterior tendon, which is commonly degenerated. Instead, the authors use the distal stump of the posterior tibialis tendon to anchor the flexor digitorum longus (FDL) tendon against it. They anchor it using a side-by-side tenorrhaphy with nonabsorbable sutures, pulling the FDL tendon distally in maximum tension.

The authors prefer this reconstruction variation over the Brodell method, because for the Brodell and colleagues' technique, an 8- to 10-mm tunnel is needed at the sustentaculum tali to be able to fit both tendon ends. For the authors' patient population, this tunnel size could jeopardize the sustentaculum tali integrity. The recommended reconstruction needs a 5-mm calcaneus tunnel, which will not weaken the sustentaculum tali structure. To the best of the authors' knowledge, Brodell and colleagues are the only investigators with published results using a tibiocalcaneonavicular ligament reconstruction.[35] They reported 12 flatfeet patients with advanced deformity that underwent the aforementioned ligament reconstruction, with a 24-month average follow-up period, showing excellent clinical outcomes and radiographic improvement.

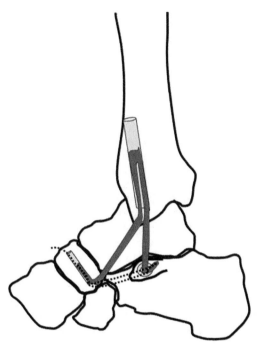

Fig. 13. The medial hindfoot, where the reconstruction of the tibiocalcaneonavicular ligament is represented. The graft is represented as a tubular structure between the tibia, sustentaculum tali, and navicular. A suture tape is represented as a dotted line structure between the sustentaculum tali and navicular.

Midfoot Instability

Bone reconstruction

When trying to pinpoint a precise apex of deformity along the medial arch, this is not possible most of the time. On weight-bearing lateral foot radiographs, a diffuse medial column sag is generally present. Addressing medial arch instability through fusions may not be the best option, as joint-preserving surgeries are preferable in flexible non-arthritic flatfoot patients. A finite element study was presented recently that showed that a naviculocuneiform fusion led to increased stress on the spring ligament, which supports the idea of avoiding fusions in this area.[36] Classically residual medial column instability has been addressed through a dorsal opening wedge osteotomy of the medial cuneiform. It has been shown that caution should be undertaken when performing this procedure, as excessive plantar flexion does not correlate with good functional outcomes.[26] Precise calculations have been published to know how much of a correction of the cuneiform morphology will be achieved with the osteotomy.[37] Relative to the last component of the medial column, that is, the tarsometatarsal joint, if there is additional involvement with a hallux valgus deformity, a tarsometatarsal arthrodesis will be an effective way of addressing both deformities.[9] If no additional deformity is present, the authors recommend performing tibiocalcaneonavicular soft tissue reconstructions to avoid fusions on the medial column. If there are imaging or intraoperative findings that suggest isolated spring ligament damage, isolated spring ligament repair can be performed.

Soft tissue reconstruction

The spring ligament repair is addressed elsewhere in this issue, and the readers are strongly encouraged to look at the corresponding article (see Caio Nery and Daniel Baumfeld's article "Current Trends in Treatment of Injuries to Spring Ligament").

Tendon transfers

Although it is not discussed in this article, for most cases where a complete medial repair is performed, a tendon transfer is recommended. Frequently, an extensive tibialis posterior tendon degeneration is present in flatfeet patients. An FDL transfer is frequently used to reinforce or to replace the tibialis posterior. The authors do not usually resect the tibialis posterior, but they do shorten it. The FDL transfer is sutured in a side-to-side fashion to the distal tibialis posterior tendon stump. The tendon transfer is performed after the tibiocalcaneonavicular reconstruction is finished.

SUMMARY

Flatfoot deformity continues to be a challenging problem. Its various clinical presentations, deformity components, and severity contribute to its complexity. The ligament incompetence responsible for this complex deformity is multifactorial, comprising morphologically different ligaments, such as the tibio-spring, tibionavicular tibiocalcaneal, and spring ligament, besides the plantar fascia and posterior tibial tendon. Recently, a more functional division of the previously named ligaments has been published, naming the whole medial ankle ligament complex as the tibiocalcaneonavicular ligament. This more global understanding of medial ankle ligaments has pushed forward investigations trying to repair or reconstruct this wide ligament complex as a unit, instead of treating individual components of it. Depending on the different apices of deformity present, flatfoot deformity should be addressed always with skeletal and soft tissue procedures.

CLINICS CARE POINTS

- Flatfoot deformity is explained by a combination of ligament insufficiencies. This fact explains the multiple apices of deformity generally present in flatfeet cases.[1]
- An isolated failure of the posterior tibial tendon is not enough to explain a flatfoot deformity.[4]
- An essential component of hindfoot malalignment is a coronal rotation of the talus over the calcaneus. This malrotation must be addressed when treating flatfoot deformities.[3]
- The medial ankle ligament complex probably works as a functional unit, with insertion points on the tibia, navicular, and calcaneus. It is called the tibiocalcaneonavicular ligament, comprising the previously named tibionavicular, tibiospring, and tibiocalcaneal ligaments.[18]
- Recent studies try to reconstruct the tibiocalcaneonavicular ligament as a complex, not as individual units.[35]

DISCLOSURE

The authors have nothing to disclose.

REFERENCES

1. Deland JT, de Asla RJ, Sung IH, et al. Posterior tibial tendon insufficiency: which ligaments are involved? Foot Ankle Int 2005;26(6):427–35.

2. Deland JT. Adult-acquired flatfoot deformity. J Am Acad Orthop Surg 2008;16(7): 399–406.
3. Kodithuwakku Arachchige SNK, Chander H, Knight A. Flatfeet: biomechanical implications, assessment, and management. Foot (Edinb) 2019;38:81–5.
4. Cifuentes-De la Portilla C, Larrainzar-Garijo R, Bayod J. Biomechanical stress analysis of the main soft tissues associated with the development of adult acquired flatfoot deformity. Clin Biomech (Bristol, Avon) 2019;61:163–71.
5. Watanabe K, Kitaoka HB, Fujii T, et al. Posterior tibial tendon dysfunction and flatfoot: analysis with simulated walking. Gait Posture 2013;37(2):264–8.
6. Arangio GA, Salathe EP. A biomechanical analysis of posterior tibial tendon dysfunction, medial displacement calcaneal osteotomy and flexor digitorum longus transfer in adult acquired flat foot. Clin Biomech (Bristol, Avon) 2009;24(4): 385–90 [published correction appears in Clin Biomech (Bristol, Avon). 2009 Jul;24(6):530].
7. Swanton E, Fisher L, Fisher A, et al. An anatomic study of the naviculocuneiform ligament and its possible role maintaining the medial longitudinal arch. Foot Ankle Int 2019;40(3):352–5.
8. Chan F, Bowlby MA, Christensen JC. Medial column biomechanics: nonsurgical and surgical implications. Clin Podiatr Med Surg 2020;37(1):39–51.
9. Kadakia AR, Kelikian AS, Barbosa M, et al. Did failure occur because of medial column instability that was not recognized, or did it develop after surgery? Foot Ankle Clin 2017;22(3):545–62.
10. Saltzman C, El-Khoury G. The hindfoot alignment view. Foot Ankle Int 1995; 16:572.
11. Paley D, Herzenberg J, Tetsworth K, et al. Deformity planning for frontal and sagittal plane corrective osteotomies. Orthop Clin North Am 1994;25(3):425–65.
12. Lopez M, Wagner P. Analisis y plan quirúrgico de deformidades en tobillo y retropié del adulto. Rev Chil Ortop Traumatol 2019. https://doi.org/10.1055/s-0039-3400508.
13. Hintermann B, Knupp M, Barg A. Joint-preserving surgery of asymmetric ankle osteoarthritis with peritalar instability. Foot Ankle Clin 2013;18(3):503–16.
14. Hintermann B, Knupp M, Barg A. Peritalar instability. Foot Ankle Int 2012;33(5): 450–4.
15. Nosewicz TL, Knupp M, Bolliger L, et al. Radiological morphology of peritalar instability in varus and valgus tilted ankles. Foot Ankle Int 2014;35(5):453–62.
16. Wang B, Saltzman CL, Chalayon O, et al. Does the subtalar joint compensate for ankle malalignment in end-stage ankle arthritis? Clin Orthop Relat Res 2015; 473(1):318–25.
17. Williamson ER, Chan JY, Burket JC, et al. New radiographic parameter assessing hindfoot alignment in stage II adult-acquired flatfoot deformity. Foot Ankle Int 2015;36(4):417–23.
18. Cromeens BP, Kirchhoff CA, Patterson RM, et al. An attachment-based description of the medial collateral and spring ligament complexes. Foot Ankle Int 2015; 36(6):710–21.
19. Masaragian HJ, Massetti S, Perin F, et al. Flatfoot deformity due to isolated spring ligament injury. J Foot Ankle Surg 2020;59(3):469–78.
20. Hintermann B. Medial ankle instability. Foot Ankle Clin 2003;8(4):723–38.
21. Kitaoka HB, Patzer GL. Subtalar arthrodesis for posterior tibial tendon dysfunction and pes planus. Clin Orthop Relat Res 1997;345:187–94.

22. Kitaoka HB, Luo ZP, An KN. Subtalar arthrodesis versus flexor digitorum longus tendon transfer for severe flatfoot deformity: an in vitro biomechanical analysis. Foot Ankle Int 1997;18(11):710–5.
23. Cohen BE, Johnson JE. Subtalar arthrodesis for treatment of posterior tibial tendon insufficiency. Foot Ankle Clin 2001;6(1):121–8.
24. Knupp M. The use of osteotomies in the treatment of asymmetric ankle joint arthritis. Foot Ankle Int 2017;38(2):220–9.
25. Vander Griend R. Lateral column lengthening using a "Z" osteotomy of the calcaneus. Tech Foot Ankle Surg 2008;7(4):257–63.
26. Conti MS, Garfinkel JH, Ellis SJ. Outcomes of reconstruction of the flexible adult-acquired flatfoot deformity. Orthop Clin North Am 2020;51(1):109–20.
27. Chan JY, Greenfield ST, Soukup DS, et al. Contribution of lateral column lengthening to correction of forefoot abduction in stage IIb adult acquired flatfoot deformity reconstruction. Foot Ankle Int 2015;36(12):1400–11.
28. Patel M, Barbosa M, Kadakia A. Role of spring and deltoid ligament reconstruction for adult acquired flatfoot deformity. Tech Foot Ankle 2017;16:124–35.
29. Huang CK, Kitaoka HB, An KN, et al. Biomechanical evaluation of longitudinal arch stability. Foot Ankle 1993;14(6):353–7.
30. Williams BR, Ellis SJ, Deyer TW, et al. Reconstruction of the spring ligament using a peroneus longus autograft tendon transfer. Foot Ankle Int 2010;31(7):567–77.
31. Xu C, Zhang MY, Lei GH, et al. Biomechanical evaluation of tenodesis reconstruction in ankle with deltoid ligament deficiency: a finite element analysis. Knee Surg Sports Traumatol Arthrosc 2012;20(9):1854–62.
32. Baxter JR, LaMothe JM, Walls RJ, et al. Reconstruction of the medial talonavicular joint in simulated flatfoot deformity. Foot Ankle Int 2015;36(4):424–9.
33. Grunfeld R, Oh I, Flemister S, et al. Reconstruction of the deltoid-spring ligament. Tech Foot Ankle Surg 2016;15(1):39–46.
34. Nery C, Lemos AVKC, Raduan F, et al. Combined spring and deltoid ligament repair in adult-acquired flatfoot. Foot Ankle Int 2018;39(8):903–7.
35. Brodell JD Jr, MacDonald A, Perkins JA, et al. Deltoid-spring ligament reconstruction in adult acquired flatfoot deformity with medial peritalar instability. Foot Ankle Int 2019;40(7):753–61.
36. Cifuentes-De la Portilla C, Pasapula C, Larrainzar-Garijo R, et al. Finite element analysis of secondary effect of midfoot fusions on the spring ligament in the management of adult acquired flatfoot [published online ahead of print, 2020 May 6]. Clin Biomech (Bristol, Avon) 2020;76:105018.
37. Kunas GC, Do HT, Aiyer A, et al. Contribution of medial cuneiform osteotomy to correction of longitudinal arch collapse in stage IIb adult-acquired flatfoot deformity. Foot Ankle Int 2018;39(8):885–93.

The Failed Deltoid Ligament in the Valgus Misaligned Ankle—How to Treat?

Norman Espinosa, MD*, Georg Klammer, MD

KEYWORDS

• Deltoid • Ligament • Failed • Therapy • Management • Solutions • Valgus • Ankle

KEY POINTS

- Failed deltoid ligament is a chronic condition.
- Chronic conditions usually are associated with insufficient tissues for reconstruction.
- Proper analysis is required before embarking on surgery.
- Nonoperative measures have a limited value in the treatment of those cases.
- Anatomic reconstructions of the medial collateral ligament complex are preferred.
- Additional surgeries are frequently needed to ensure a successful outcome.

INTRODUCTION

The medial collateral ligament around the ankle, that is, the deltoid ligament, is the primary stabilizer of the ankle joint.[1] Therefore, its role for hindfoot biomechanics is of pivotal importance. Chronic deltoid injuries as well as insufficiencies are challenging for the orthopedic foot and ankle surgeon. If left untreated, any incompetence of the medial ligamentous apparatus ends up in chronic pain, rotational instability, and hindfoot deformity, which in turn accelerate progressive hindfoot degeneration, that is, osteoarthritis.[2] Once osteoarthritis has taken place in association with an unstable deltoid ligament, it becomes difficult to manage by total ankle arthroplasty (TAA), and, in some cases, fusions remain the only treatment options. Thus, any falsely treated deltoid ligament pathology may preclude certain essential treatment strategies, which would fare much better than a functionally impairing strategy.

    This article deals with the chronically failed deltoid ligament in the valgus misaligned ankle. A proper analysis is crucial and should be done as a first step before embarking on any treatment in those specific cases. This helps select the adequate treatment option, avoid new problems, and gain a certain impression of the future prognosis for the function and integrity of the ankle joint.

Institute for Foot and Ankle Reconstruction, Beethovenstrasse 3, Zurich 8002, Switzerland
* Corresponding author.
E-mail address: espinosa@fussinstitut.ch

Foot Ankle Clin N Am 26 (2021) 391–405
https://doi.org/10.1016/j.fcl.2021.03.011
1083-7515/21/© 2021 Elsevier Inc. All rights reserved.

BIOMECHANICAL THOUGHTS ON DELTOID LIGAMENT FUNCTION

As discussed previously, the role of the deltoid ligament is essential for the medial stability of the ankle. Its integrity prevents lateral translation and valgus angulation of the hindfoot.[3–5]

The superficial layer limits external rotation and valgus stress at the ankle joint. The deep layer limits ankle eversion and lateral translation of talus. Thus, lesions of the deep deltoid layer tend to cause lateral and anterior displacement of the talus, whereas superficial lesions may not result in translation but increased valgus moment at the ankle joint, especially when the tibiocalcaneal bundle is involved.[4] In cadaveric model studies, deltoid ligament sectioning led to 15% to 20% decrease in ankle joint contact area.[6] Other studies were able to demonstrate that superficial deltoid ligament sectioning resulted in reduction of ankle contact area up to 43%.[7–9]

ANALYSIS OF THE FAILED DELTOID LIGAMENT

It is important to distinguish primary and structural failure of the deltoid ligament from secondary failure due to chronic overload subsequent to neglected pathologies that result in attenuation and incompetence of medial ankle ligaments.

Primary Structural Injury of the Deltoid Ligament

The deltoid ligament can be injured by a wide pattern of direct lesions starting from partial and ending up in complete tears of the tissue. Most common might be the association with ankle sprains, a direct hit, penetrating trauma, or ankle fractures. All of these cause local damage to the deltoid ligament, which causes instability of variable extent.

Eversion and external rotation of the ankle stresses the deltoid ligament complex. In fractures, the supination external rotation IV and pronation external rotation III/IV types disrupt the deltoid ligament complex.[10,11]

Several scientific articles state that it is not necessary to fix the deltoid ligament in the acute setting of fractures.[12] These, however, also may become causes of chronic medial ankle instability. This findings may might be true for missed syndesmotic lesions, where a lateral shift of the talus starts to involve the medial collateral ligament complex.[11]

Secondary Structural Injury of the Deltoid Ligament

Secondary structural injury of the deltoid ligament is a more complex entity. Inadequate treatment of chronic ankle instability as a sequel of an ankle sprain can lead to local overload of the superficial bundles of the deltoid ligament, which—over time—starts to stretch out, increasing the valgus moment within the ankle mortise.[13,14]

Insufficiency of the posterior tibial tendon with consecutive alteration of the muscle function can cause chronic overload of the deltoid ligament. This is due mainly to the valgus and pronatory moment at the hindfoot under foot loading.[13]

Fixed hindfoot valgus misalignment and flatfoot deformities may lead to secondary failure of the tibiocalcaneal bundles of the deltoid ligament.

Forefoot-driven hindfoot valgus is a flexible deformity due to an instability of the medial ray. Unfortunately, there is no evidence of such a pathology found in the literature. In the authors' experience, however, it does exist. As a result of an unstable medial column, the pronation of the hindfoot exerts forces along the medial hindfoot, including the subtalar joint, resulting in chronic overload of the deltoid ligament structure.

PREPARING TO SOLVE THE PROBLEM OF A FAILED DELTOID LIGAMENT

It is essential to prepare properly before embarking on deltoid ligament repair. This is because in various cases not only does the ligament need to be reconstructed but also additional surgeries must be considered to ensure full correction of the deformity and long-term stability.

The process of preparation includes clinical assessment, imaging, and selection of treatment (conservative vs surgical).

Functional Evaluation of the Medial Collateral Ligament Complex

This is a brief overview focusing specifically on the assessment of the deltoid ligament; medial column, including the collateral ligament complex; and posterior tibial tendon function.

Normally, a patient is examined in standing and sitting positions. During standing, the hindfoot is examined visually from posterior. The amount of valgus deformity can be measured using the intersection between the midline of the Achilles tendon and the midline of the calcaneus. Any prominence of the medial malleolus needs to be identified. As a valuable test, the patient is requested to actively correct the hindfoot valgus into neutral. This indicates an intact posterior tibial tendon function and raises the probability of deltoid ligament and/or spring ligament incompetence. Hintermann and Gächter[15] were able to show that with an external rotation of the shank the heel can be brought into varus. In cases of a dysfunctional posterior tibial tendon, the first metatarsal head is elevated, whereas it remains on ground, if normal. Additionally, the single heel-rise test helps to evaluate the integrity of the posterior tibial tendon function.[16]

In order to assess any forefoot-driven hindfoot valgus, the authors use the so-called reversed Coleman block test (**Fig. 1**). This is done while placing a support underneath

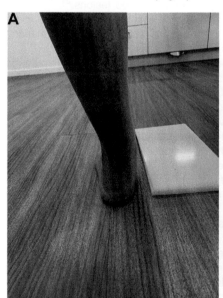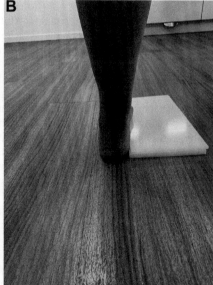

Fig. 1. (*A*) The figure shows the patient standing in front of the physician without any support. Note the hindfoot valgus. (*B*) The same patient depicted with a medial support underneath the first ray. The hindfoot has corrected into neutral.

the heel and the first ray. When the hindfoot corrects into neutral, the diagnosis is confirmed. In addition, manual testing for any hypermobility of the first ray should be done.[17–19]

In the sitting position, the foot is palpated to identify any tenderness at the medial gutter or along the course of the posterior tibial tendon and spring ligament. External rotation can be used to stress the deltoid ligament. In addition, external rotation and eversion may be applied for gross assessment of medial ankle instability. Similar to lateral ankle instability, an anterior drawer test might be applied.[20] In cases of chronic rotational ankle instability, however, it might be difficult to distinguish between lateral and medial ligamentous incompetence.

Assessment of muscle strength is mandatory, specifically when tendon transfers are taken into consideration.

Imaging Techniques to Assess Deltoid Ligament Incompetence

Standard weight-bearing foot and ankle radiographs are needed to assess any deformity at the hindfoot and possible lesions.

Those include

- Anteroposterior, mortise views
- Lateral views
- Dorsoplantar views
- Hindfoot alignment views: Saltzman view[21] or long axial views (less susceptible to rotation and, therefore, preferred by the authors)[22,23]
- Full-leg views to assess the position of the knee and hip

Conventional radiographs allow assessment of structural valgus deformities taking place at the hindfoot, midfoot, and forefoot and whether arthrosis is present or not.

Magnetic resonance imaging (MRI) has become widely accepted and an accurate modality to assess the soft tissues, cartilage, and associated lesions.[24–28] But Yu and colleagues[29] also were able to show that, in the acute setting, 20% false-negative MRI findings were obtained. This indicates the high difficulty of evaluating the chronic conditions of deltoid insufficiency.[29]

The superficial deltoid tear might be found at its insertion slightly proximal to the tip of the medial malleolus. It is seen best on coronal images. Deep deltoid ligament lesions and spring ligament lesions also can be identified on coronal images.[20] Usually, in deep deltoid lesions, the feathering aspect of the structure is lost. Sometimes avulsion can be seen. It may be blurred, however, in larger lesions.[24,30–32]

Ultrasound has become a useful tool in the assessment of ligament lesions. In acute lesions, ultrasound has shown a sensitivity of almost 94% and 100% specificity compared with MRI.[33,34] One of the greatest advantages of ultrasound over MRI is the possibility of functional in vivo testing of the hindfoot structures. Ultrasound, however, always is operator-dependent. Thus, a lot of experience is required to interpret the results of the examination properly.

Weightbearing-CT (WBCT)has become a novel and effectice tool for the assessment of hindfoot deformities.[35] Burssens and colleagues presented a method of measuring the angular deformities.[36] One of the greatest advantages of WBCT is to assess pathological deformities under loading conditions. This enables a better insight into the deformity and where it might take place, which in turns allows a more accurate planning for corrections. More recently, the a consensus group statement has been published voting in favour to use the WBCT as a part of the classification system and strongly voted for its use in the preoperative planning in patients suffering from progressive flatfoot deformity.[37,38] However, up to now, not every surgeon/clinic might have access to this technology. Therefore, most surgeons may be adhere to the formerly mentioned imaging techniques. Besides this, there are still further studies needed to to draw better conclusions of how to apply this technique for all entire hind-foot deformities. According to the opinion of the authors this technique has its huge merits in the assessment of flatfoot deformities.

TREATMENT OF THE CHRONICALLY FAILED DELTOID LIGAMENT

When deciding to treat a failed deltoid ligament complex in the presence of a valgus ankle, it is essential to answer the following question: Is the repair/reconstruction of the deltoid feasible or not?

In many patients who suffer from chronically failed deltoid ligament function, the iso-lated repair of the deltoid might not be sufficient enough to cope with the integral dysfunction of the hindfoot. Thus, a surgeon needs to evaluate the pathology properly and find the optimal solution.

In general, it can be expected that, in chronic failures of the deltoid ligament, struc-tural deficiencies have taken place, which in turn complicate the entire treatment.

Conservative Treatment

Nonoperative treatment strategies are reserved for minimal deformities and patients who are not candidates for surgery due to medical reasons.

Physical therapy tries to improve coordination and proprioception. In addition, physical therapy helps increase muscle strength for better hindfoot control.[39–42]

In patients with minimal and flexible hindfoot valgus insoles, providing a medial arch support with or without heel support may help correct the position of the foot and improve postural control (due to increased plantar cutaneous feedback).[43] Sometimes taping may help improve the outcome.

Braces, which are designed to resist loads in the transversal and coronal plane, can augment stability by neurologic feedback through cutaneous and mechanoreceptors. Patients should wear the braces for a minimum of 6 months until deciding whether or not surgery is warranted.[44–47]

Specific and tailored shoes are required for patients who are not easy to control regarding deformity, who refuse surgical treatment, and who are medically very ill.

Surgical Treatment

The literature reveals several techniques to repair the deltoid ligament complex. The authors provide their own algorithm of failed deltoid ligament management, which is based on the data available in the literature and on their own experience.

Chronic failures reveal an impaired structural integrity of the ligamentous complex jeopardizing any surgical treatment. The surgical strategy should take this fact into ac-count and try to optimize outcome.

Anatomic deltoid ligament reconstruction

The first author has adopted and modified the techniques described by Haddad and colleagues[48] and Nery and colleagues[49] (**Figs. 2** and **3**). Both techniques allow an anatomic reconstruction of the deltoid ligament, including the option to repair the spring ligament where needed. Originally described with the use of tendon grafts, the same method can be performed utilizing nonresorbable fiber sutures.[50]

The deltoid ligament is approached from posteromedial. The incision is made slightly dorsal to the edge of the course of the posterior tibial tendon. After careful sub-cutaneous preparation, the sheath covering the posterior tibial tendon is exposed and opened. The posterior tibial tendon becomes visible and can be moved plantarly by

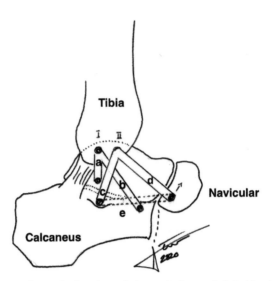

Fig. 2. Depicted is a schematic drawing of the technique of deltoid +/- spring ligament repair as discussed in text: a, tibiotalar ligament reconstruction; b, tibiospring reconstruction; c, tibiocalcaneal reconstruction; d, tibiospring reconstruction; and e, additional spring ligament reconstruction in case of a complete rupture of the spring ligament.

means of a Langenbeck hook. At this stage of the procedure, the deltoid ligament and spring ligament as well can be identified. The navicular tuberosity (dorsal to the insertion of the posterior tibial tendon) and sustentaculum tali both need to be exposed. Care should be taken to not injure the tendon of the flexor digitorum longus or flexor hallucis longus. In addition, the anterior and medial parts of the calcaneus as well as the tip of the medial malleolus need to be exposed. Two drill holes are made in the medial malleolus. Two autologous or allografts (minor morbidity) are needed for the reconstruction. Alternatively, new tools, for example, the InternalBrace (Arthrex; Naples, Florida), can be used. Additional drill holes are made in the navicular tuberosity, anteromedial part of the calcaneus, and sustentaculum tali.

The first graft is inserted with 1 end into the medial surface of the talus and secured with an interference screw. The foot is held in neutral position. Then the graft is brought close to the inferior drill hole in the medial malleolus and its limbed secured by means of an interference screw. This reconstructs the tibiotalar ligament. Afterward, the distal graft limb is inserted into the drill hole, which has been made in the anteromedial portion of the calcaneus and passed from medial to lateral to achieve proper tension. The graft then is secured by means of an additional interference screw. This part reconstructs the tibiospring ligament.

The second graft then is inserted with 1 end into the sustentaculum tali and secured with an interference screw. The distal part of the graft is then inserted into the anterior drill hole of the medial malleolus and secured. This reconstruction creates a band that connects the tibia and calcaneus. It corresponds to the tibiocalcaneal ligament and enhances the construct. Then the rest of the graft can be inserted, under tension, within the navicular tuberosity and fixed with an interference screw. This last step reconstructs the tibionavicular ligament.

By doing so, the surgical technique allows the reconstruction of 4 ligaments. In cases of a complete rupture of the spring ligament, an additional graft/suture might be used, which is driven from the navicular tuberosity to the sustentaculum tali.

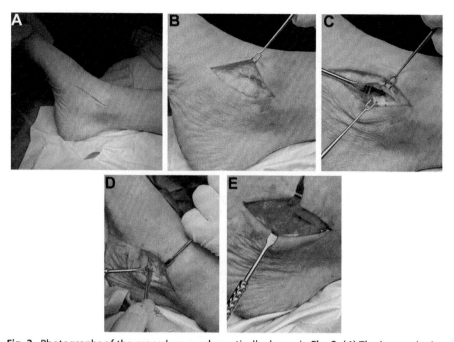

Fig. 3. Photographs of the procedure as schematically drawn in **Fig. 2.** (*A*) The image depicts the skin incision for the approach. This is done posteromedially just at the dorsal edge of the course of the posterior tibial tendon. (*B*) After careful subcutaneous dissection, the posterior tibial tendon sheath is exposed and incised. (*C*) The image shows the intraoperative finding of the chronically failed deltoid ligament. In the depth of the lesion the medial wall of the talus can be appreciated. The tip of the medial malleolus shows irregularities without any sign of ligamentous attachment. (*D*) This photograph shows how to access the anterior and medial part of the calcaneus. The posterior tibial tendon is intact and reflected plantarly in order to get access to the calcaneus. (*E*) Final result after the procedure. The tibionavicular ligament reconstruction is tightened because of the plantarflexed position of the hindfoot. In contrast, in neutral or dorsal position of the hindfoot, the reconstructed tibiotalar (deep portion), tibiocalcaneal, and tibiospring ligament become tightened whereas the tibionaviculare strand relaxes somewhat. The entire construct finally is stabilized by suturing the remnants of the ligaments onto the fiber strands.

Unfeasible reconstruction

When there is no way to reconstruct the deltoid ligament complex, the only solution that can be considered is tibiotalar or tibiotalocalcaneal fusion.

ADDITIONAL SURGERIES

In chronic deltoid ligament failure, it often is necessary to add further surgical treatments. In addition, if chronic deltoid injury is a secondary result of a certain pathology, the primary and driving forces needs to be addressed. The goal of additional surgeries is to protect the final reconstruction of the deltoid ligament complex.

Lateral Ligament Reconstruction

In cases of chronic rotational hindfoot instability found, the lateral ligament complex should be reconstructed. This can be done either by a simple Broström procedure[51,52] (viable ligament tissue needed) or reconstruction by means of tendon graft use.[53]

Medializing Calcaneal Osteotomy

A medializing calcaneal osteotomy alters the pulling vector of the Achilles tendon. As a result of it, the subtalar joint also is corrected and the reconstruction of the medial collateral complex protected. When there is doubt regarding the long-term result after deltoid ligament reconstruction and if there is still a remaining hindfoot valgus left, the medializing calcaneal osteotomy offers reasonable stability to the hindfoot.[1,54–56]

Evans and Hintermann Osteotomy—Lateral Column Lengthening Procedures

In certain cases of forefoot abduction, it might be necessary to add a lateral calcaneal lengthening procedure to rotate and swing the Chopart joint around the coronal and transversal planes.[57]

Flexor Digitorum Transfer

A transfer of the flexor digitorum longus is needed in the presence of a dysfunctional posterior tibial tendon. This procedure often is done in combination with a medializing calcaneal osteotomy.[58,59]

Supramalleolar Osteotomies

In patients with a valgus hindfoot deformity that is caused not only by an insufficient deltoid ligament complex but also by deformity of the distal lower leg, supramalleolar osteotomies might be added. In congruent types, dome osteotomies may be considered, whereas in incongruent types, lateral closing wedge or medial opening wedge osteotomies could be performed.[60–62]

Medial Column Fusion

In cases of forefoot-driven hindfoot valgus (with hypermobility of the medial column), it might be necessary to perform a first tarsometatarsal, naviculocuneiform, or combined fusion. The site of correction depends on the apex of deformity found in the preoperative assessment.

Naviculocuneiform and Subtalar Fusion

In an attempt to avoid too much hindfoot stiffness Steiner and colleagues presented the fusion of the naviculocuneifom joint in combination with a talonavicular fusion.[63] The procedure leaves the Chopart-joint open and flexible while ensuring a durable result in patient with flatfoot deformity.

An other way to correct specific flatfoot deformities is to fuse the subtalar joint.[64] The procedure is considered helpful in patients who present with lateral ankle pain, e.g. sinus tarsi impingement and in even worse cases, subfibular impingement due to stiff flatfoot deformity. These pathologies can be seen as subsequent results of a so-called peritalar subluxation. Therefore, in order to prevent a failure of the reconstruction, it might not be preferable to salvage the subtalar joint but rather to fuse it while correcting the peritalar deformity.[65]

Diple Arthrodesis

The use of a diple arthrodesis (subtalar and talonavicular fusion) is warranted when arthritic changes already have taken place in the subtalar and Chopart joint and when rigid valgus deformities are encountered that preclude any joint-preserving technique.[65,66]

Syndesmotic Reconstruction

Syndesmotic reconstruction is mandatory when the fibula and talus both shift laterally while the ankle tilts into valgus. The first author uses a modified technique based on Morris and colleagues'[67] description of syndesmotic repair. As an alternative, special suture techniques can be used. In chronic cases, the necessity of autograft or allograft tendons for reconstruction should be considered. Vila-Rico and colleagues[68] presented an anatomic arthroscopic graft reconstruction for chronic disruption of the distal syndesmosis. The technique, which is performed minimally invasively, seems to have its merit. As an alternative, syndesmotic fusion can be performed. Fusion might be problematic, however, and requires additional autologous or allogeneic bone graft.

THOUGHTS ON TOTAL ANKLE ARTHROPLASTY IN A VALGUS ANKLE

When considering a TAA in a valgus ankle joint, it is important to follow a logical algorithm or path in order to achieve a stable implantation. Perfect balance of a TAA ensures longevity of the implant and great success of the procedure.

Before embarking on such a procedure, it is mandatory to identify the type of valgus deformity. This article does not discuss supramalleolar deformity aspects.

When planning to implant a TAA in a valgus ankle, the authors follow 4 criteria:

1. The fibula

    A short fibula may lead to a valgus moment within the ankle joint. As a consequence, the talus tilts into valgus and may exert too much stress onto the deltoid ligament, which in turn starts to stretch out resulting in progressive insufficiency.

    Solution: consider lengthening of the fibula.[69]
2. The syndesmosis

    Any unstable syndesmosis may result in a lateral shift of the talus. As a result, the deltoid ligament becomes stretched and potentially incompetent.

    Solution: consider either anatomic reconstruction by a graft or fusion.[67,70,71]
3. Lateral distal tibial plafond (**Fig. 4**)

    In a long-standing valgus ankle, the talus may start to erode the lateral distal tibial surface. By doing so, the valgus moment increases, leading to increased pull onto the deltoid ligament, which may deteriorate continuously over time.

    Solution: correction through tibial cut and use of so-called spacer effect of the polyethylene inlay.[61]
4. Deltoid ligament integrity

    In cases of valgus deformity, it might be that the deltoid is insufficient. Whenever the deltoid becomes insufficient, the surgeon needs to verify whether this is a relative issue due to overlength caused by other causes or because it is structurally damaged. The latter case is worse than the former, as discussed later.

    Solutions: direct repair using reefing sutures and/or anchors/anatomic reconstruction using graft tissue or specific implants.

These criteria can be present as combinations. Thus, it is important to look for those and to address the problems accurately.

The structural integrity of the deltoid ligament is assessed clinically and verified by MRI. The main question is whether the deltoid ligament shows viable structural value

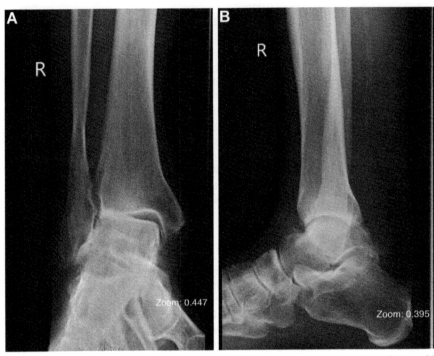

Fig. 4. The image shows the (A) anterior and (B) lateral radiographs of a valgus ankle arthritis. The talus tilts into valgus and has a close contact with the fibula, which represents a normal length. There is an erosion of the lateral distal tibial plafond and a slight medial joint gap.

or if it is severely impaired. In cases of a severely lesioned deltoid ligament, the authors do not perform a TAA and prefer an ankle arthrodesis.

When viable tissue is present, however, surgeons may consider a repair, which could be done in either a 1-staged or 2-staged fashion.

One-staged Total Ankle Arthroplasty Implantation (With Specific Regard to Deltoid Incompetence)

In order to assess the correction of valgus deformity during surgery, it is appropriate to use a spreader, which is placed laterally over the tibia and talus. When opening the spreader, the valgus deformity may be corrected. If it is possible to put both articular surfaces parallel to each other, the deformity can be corrected by the tibial cut and through the so-called spacer effect of the polyethylene inlay (see **Fig. 4; Fig. 5**).[61] This is an appropriate way to correct the valgus deformity.

In cases of subtle deltoid lesions causing medial ankle instability, a reefing of the deltoid ligament might be considered. This kind of procedure resembles more a Broström-technique rather than a true reconstruction.[12,72,73]

Two-staged Total Ankle Arthroplasty Implantation (With Specific Regard to Deltoid Incompetence)

Any other lesion and major damage, for example, severe deltoid incompetence, should be treated by a 2-staged procedure. The technique, as described in this article, can be considered to restore the anatomy and biomechanical integrity of the medial collateral ligament complex. After such a reconstruction, however, the surgeon should

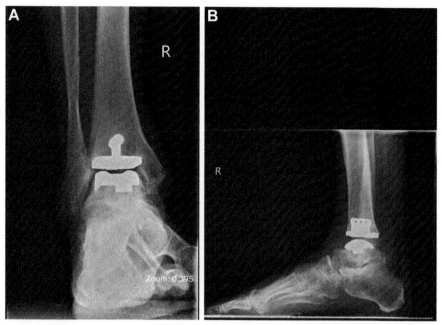

Fig. 5. Depicted are the postoperative (*A*) anterior and (*B*) lateral views of the same patients described in **Fig. 4**, 2 years postoperatively. It easily can be appreciated how the spacer effect has worked. Correction of the valgus has been achieved through the tibial cut and spanning of the polyethylene inlay.

be sure that the medial ankle part has become stable. Once this is achieved, the TAA can be planned. Additional procedures, as discussed previously, need to be taken into consideration.

If the deltoid is not repaired properly and an instability persists, it is highly probable that the TAA will fail.[74,75]

OUTCOMES OF DELTOID RECONSTRUCTION IN THE LITERATURE

Hintermann and colleagues[43] reported on the results after surgical reconstruction of medial collateral ligament complex. The found, at an average follow-up of 4.43 years (2–6.5 years) after surgical reconstruction, good to excellent clinical results in 46 cases (90%), fair in 4 cases (8%), and poor in 1 case (2%).

More recently, Pellegrini and colleagues[76] published their results of deltoid ligament repair by an InternalBrace augmentation. For their study, 13 patients were included. After a mean follow-up of 13.5. months, the patients revealed good results. Of these, 2 implant failures were recorded without apparent compromise of construct stability.

Quite good results also have been reported by Nery and colleagues.[49] The group presented their results of a combined surgical repair of the deltoid and spring ligament in 10 patients. At a mean follow-up of 20 months, all patients were able to perform the single heel-rise test while the average functional result score was 86 points in the American Orthopaedic Foot and Ankle Society scale.

SUMMARY

Reconstruction of a chronically failed deltoid ligament complex in a valgus misaligned hindfoot is demanding. It requires a proper preoperative plan in order to achieve a successful result. Among the variety of techniques published in the contemporary scientific literature, anatomic reconstructions are preferred.

An orthopedic foot and ankle surgeon needs to be aware that not only the ligament reconstruction but also additional surgeries need to be done to ensure a good functional outcome.

DISCLOSURE

The authors have nothing to disclose.

REFERENCES

1. Hintermann B. Medial ankle instability. Foot Ankle Clin 2003;8(4):723–38.
2. Abdulazim AN, Horisberger M, Knupp M. [Medial foot and ankle instability]. Unfallchirurg 2019;122(2):147–59.
3. Bastias GF, Dalmau-Pastor M, Astudillo C, et al. Spring Ligament Instability. Foot Ankle Clin 2018;23(4):659–78.
4. Harper MC. The deltoid ligament. An evaluation of need for surgical repair. Clin Orthop Relat Res 1988;(226):156–68.
5. Ferran NA, Oliva F, Maffulli N. Ankle instability. Sports Med Arthrosc 2009;17(2):139–45.
6. Clarke HJ, Michelson JD, Cox QG, et al. Tibio-talar stability in bimalleolar ankle fractures: a dynamic in vitro contact area study. Foot Ankle 1991;11(4):222–7.
7. Ellis SJ, Williams BR, Wagshul AD, et al. Deltoid ligament reconstruction with peroneus longus autograft in flatfoot deformity. Foot Ankle Int 2010;31(9):781–9.
8. Michelson JD, Clarke HJ, Jinnah RH. The effect of loading on tibiotalar alignment in cadaver ankles. Foot Ankle 1990;10(5):280–4.
9. Michelson JD, Varner KE, Checcone M. Diagnosing deltoid injury in ankle fractures: the gravity stress view. Clin Orthop Relat Res 2001;(387):178–82.
10. Hogan MV, Dare DM, Deland JT. Is deltoid and lateral ligament reconstruction necessary in varus and valgus ankle osteoarthritis, and how should these procedures be performed? Foot Ankle Clin 2013;18(3):517–27.
11. Butler BA, Hempen EC, Barbosa M, et al. Deltoid ligament repair reduces and stabilizes the talus in unstable ankle fractures. J Orthop 2020;17:87–90.
12. Lee S, Lin J, Hamid KS, et al. Deltoid ligament rupture in ankle fracture: diagnosis and management. J Am Acad Orthop Surg 2019;27(14):e648–58.
13. Boss AP, Hintermann B. Anatomical study of the medial ankle ligament complex. Foot Ankle Int 2002;23(6):547–53.
14. Hintermann B, Knupp M, Pagenstert GI. Deltoid ligament injuries: diagnosis and management. Foot Ankle Clin 2006;11(3):625–37.
15. Hintermann B, Gächter A. The first metatarsal rise sign: a simple, sensitive sign of tibialis posterior tendon dysfunction. Foot Ankle Int 1996;17(4):236–41.
16. Arain A, Harrington MC, Rosenbaum AJ. Adult Acquired flatfoot (AAFD). Treasure Island (FL: StatPearls; 2020.
17. Myerson MS, Badekas A. Hypermobility of the first ray. Foot Ankle Clin 2000;5(3):469–84.
18. Roukis TS, Landsman AS. Hypermobility of the first ray: a critical review of the literature. J Foot Ankle Surg 2003;42(6):377–90.
19. Cowie S, Parsons S, Scammell B, et al. Hypermobility of the first ray in patients with planovalgus feet and tarsometatarsal osteoarthritis. Foot Ankle Surg 2012;18(4):237–40.

20. Alshalawi S, Galhoum AE, Alrashidi Y, et al. Medial ankle instability: the deltoid dilemma. Foot Ankle Clin 2018;23(4):639–57.

21. Saltzman CL, el-Khoury GY. The hindfoot alignment view. Foot Ankle Int 1995; 16(9):572–6.

22. Buck FM, Hoffmann A, Mamisch-Saupe N, et al. Hindfoot alignment measurements: rotation-stability of measurement techniques on hindfoot alignment view and long axial view radiographs. AJR Am J Roentgenol 2011;197(3):578–82.

23. Sutter R, Pfirrmann CW, Espinosa N, et al. Three-dimensional hindfoot alignment measurements based on biplanar radiographs: comparison with standard radiographic measurements. Skeletal Radiol 2013;42(4):493–8.

24. Zanetti M. Founder's lecture of the ISS 2006: borderlands of normal and early pathological findings in MRI of the foot and ankle. Skeletal Radiol 2008;37(10): 875–84.

25. Jeong MS, Choi YS, Kim YJ, et al. Deltoid ligament in acute ankle injury: MR imaging analysis. Skeletal Radiol 2014;43(5):655–63.

26. Crim J, Longenecker LG. MRI and surgical findings in deltoid ligament tears. AJR Am J Roentgenol 2015;204(1):W63–9.

27. van Putte-Katier N, van Ochten JM, van Middelkoop M, et al. Magnetic resonance imaging abnormalities after lateral ankle trauma in injured and contralateral ankles. Eur J Radiol 2015;84(12):2586–92.

28. Salat P, Le V, Veljkovic A, et al. Imaging in foot and ankle instability. Foot Ankle Clin 2018;23(4):499.e28.

29. Yu GR, Zhang MZ, Aiyer A, et al. Repair of the acute deltoid ligament complex rupture associated with ankle fractures: a multicenter clinical study. J Foot Ankle Surg 2015;54(2):198–202.

30. Zanetti M, De Simoni C, Hodler J. [Magnetic resonance tomography (MRI) of ligament injuries of the upper ankle joint]. Sportverletz Sportschaden 1996;10(3): 58–62.

31. Mengiardi B, Pinto C, Zanetti M. Medial collateral ligament complex of the ankle: MR imaging anatomy and findings in medial instability. Semin Musculoskelet Radiol 2016;20(1):91–103.

32. Mengiardi B, Pinto C, Zanetti M. Spring ligament complex and posterior tibial tendon: MR anatomy and findings in acquired adult flatfoot deformity. Semin Musculoskelet Radiol 2016;20(1):104–15.

33. Peetrons PA, Silvestre A, Cohen M, et al. Ultrasonography of ankle ligaments. Can Assoc Radiol J 2002;53(1):6–13.

34. Henari S, Banks LN, Radovanovic I, et al. Ultrasonography as a diagnostic tool in assessing deltoid ligament injury in supination external rotation fractures of the ankle. Orthopedics 2011;34(10):e639–43.

35. Hirschmann A, Pfirrmann CW, Klammer G, et al. Upright cone CT of the hindfoot: comparison of the non-weight-bearing with the upright weight-bearing position. Eur Radiol 2014;24(3):553–8.

36. Burssens ABM, Buedts K, Barg A, et al. Is lower-limb alignment associated with hindfoot deformity in the coronal plane? a weightbearing CT analysis. Clin Orthop Relat Res 2020;478(1):154–68.

37. Myerson MS, et al. Classification and Nomenclature: Progressive Collapsing Foot Deformity. Foot Ankle Int 2020;41(10):1271–6.

38. de Cesar Netto C, et al. Consensus for the Use of Weightbearing CT in the Assessment of Progressive Collapsing Foot Deformity. Foot Ankle Int 2020; 41(10):1277–82.

39. Valderrabano V, Leumann A, Pagenstert G, et al. [Chronic ankle instability in sports – a review for sports physicians]. Sportverletz Sportschaden 2006;20(4): 177–83.

40. Ross SE, Arnold BL, Blackburn JT, et al. Enhanced balance associated with coordination training with stochastic resonance stimulation in subjects with functional ankle instability: an experimental trial. J Neuroeng Rehabil 2007;4:47.

41. Rammelt S, Schneiders W, Grass R, et al. [Ligamentous injuries to the ankle joint]. Z Orthop Unfall 2011;149(5):e45–67.

42. Weerasekara I, Osmotherly P, Snodgrass S, et al. Clinical benefits of joint mobilization on ankle sprains: a systematic review and meta-analysis. Arch Phys Med Rehabil 2018;99(7):1395.e5.

43. Hintermann B, Valderrabano V, Boss A, et al. Medial ankle instability: an exploratory, prospective study of fifty-two cases. Am J Sports Med 2004;32(1):183–90.

44. Baier M, Hopf T. Ankle orthoses effect on single-limb standing balance in athletes with functional ankle instability. Arch Phys Med Rehabil 1998;79(8):939–44.

45. Schuberth JM, Bouche RT, Reilly CH, et al. A semirigid ankle brace for chronic ankle instability. J Am Podiatry Assoc 1982;72(12):611–6.

46. Dewar RA, Arnold GP, Wang W, et al. The effects of wearing an Ankle Stabilizing Orthosis (ASO) Ankle Brace on ankle joints kinetics and kinematics during a basketball rebounding task. Foot (Edinb) 2019;40:34–8.

47. Agres AN, Chrysanthou M, Raffalt PC. The effect of ankle bracing on kinematics in simulated sprain and drop landings: a double-blind, placebo-controlled study. Am J Sports Med 2019;47(6):1480–7.

48. Haddad SL, Dedhia S, Ren Y, et al. Deltoid ligament reconstruction: a novel technique with biomechanical analysis. Foot Ankle Int 2010;31(7):639–51.

49. Nery C, Lemos AVKC, Raduan F, et al. Combined Spring and Deltoid Ligament Repair in Adult-Acquired Flatfoot. Foot Ankle Int 2018;39(8):903–7.

50. Acevedo JI, Kreulen C, Cedeno AA, et al. Technique for arthroscopic deltoid ligament repair with description of safe zones. Foot Ankle Int 2020;41(5):605–11.

51. Lee JH, Lee SH, Jung HW, et al. Modified Broström procedure in patients with chronic ankle instability is superior to conservative treatment in terms of muscle endurance and postural stability. Knee Surg Sports Traumatol Arthrosc 2020; 28(1):93–9.

52. Javors JR, Violet JT. Correction of chronic lateral ligament instability of the ankle by use of the Broström procedure. A report of 15 cases. Clin Orthop Relat Res 1985;(198):201–7.

53. Brambilla L, Bianchi A, Malerba F, et al. Lateral ankle ligament anatomic reconstruction for chronic ankle instability: Allograft or autograft? A systematic review. Foot Ankle Surg 2020;26(1):85–93.

54. Sizensky JA, Marks RM. Medial-sided bony procedures: why, what, and how? Foot Ankle Clin 2003;8(3):539–62.

55. Guha AR, Perera AM. Calcaneal osteotomy in the treatment of adult acquired flatfoot deformity. Foot Ankle Clin 2012;17(2):247–58.

56. Hamel J. [Calcaneal Z osteotomy for correction of subtalar hindfoot varus deformity]. Oper Orthop Traumatol 2015;27(4):308–16.

57. Hintermann B. [Lateral column lengthening osteotomy of calcaneus]. Oper Orthop Traumatol 2015;27(4):298–307.

58. DiDomenico LA, Thomas ZM, Fahim R. Addressing stage II posterior tibial tendon dysfunction: biomechanically repairing the osseous structures without the need of performing the flexor digitorum longus transfer. Clin Podiatr Med Surg 2014; 31(3):391–404.

59. Hentges MJ, Moore KR, Catanzariti AR, et al. Procedure selection for the flexible adult acquired flatfoot deformity. Clin Podiatr Med Surg 2014;31(3):363–79.

60. Hintermann B, Knupp M, Barg A. [Osteotomies of the distal tibia and hindfoot for ankle realignment]. Orthopade 2008;37(3):212–3, 220–3.

61. Pagenstert G, Knupp M, Valderrabano V, et al. Realignment surgery for valgus ankle osteoarthritis. Oper Orthop Traumatol 2009;21(1):77–87.

62. Hintermann B, Knupp M, Barg A. Joint-preserving surgery of asymmetric ankle osteoarthritis with peritalar instability. Foot Ankle Clin 2013;18(3):503–16.

63. Steiner CS, Gilgen A, Zwicky L, et al. Combined subtalar and naviculocuneiform fusion for treating adult acquired flatfoot deformity with medial arch collapse at the level of the naviculocuneiform joint. Foot Ankle Int 2019;40(1):42–7.

64. Hintermann B, et al. Consensus on Indications for Isolated Subtalar Joint Fusion and Naviculocuneiform Fusions for Progressive Collapsing Foot Deformity. Foot Ankle Int 2020;41(10):1295–8.

65. Knupp M, Stufkens SA, Hintermann B. Triple arthrodesis. Foot Ankle Clin 2011; 16(1):61–7.

66. Knupp M, Zwicky L, Lang TH, et al. Medial approach to the subtalar joint: anatomy, indications, technique tips. Foot Ankle Clin 2015;20(2):311–8.

67. Morris MW, Rice P, Schneider TE. Distal tibiofibular syndesmosis reconstruction using a free hamstring autograft. Foot Ankle Int 2009;30(6):506–11.

68. Vila-Rico J, Cabestany-Castellà JM, Cabestany-Perich B, et al. All-inside arthroscopic allograft reconstruction of the anterior talo-fibular ligament using an accesory transfibular portal. Foot Ankle Surg 2019;25(1):24–30.

69. Ye MY, Vaughn J, Briceno J, et al. Screw distraction technique for gaining fibular length. Injury 2018;49(12):2322–5.

70. Connors JC, Grossman JP, Zulauf EE, et al. Syndesmotic ligament allograft reconstruction for treatment of chronic diastasis. J Foot Ankle Surg 2020;59(4): 835–40.

71. Grass R, Rammelt S, Biewener A, et al. Peroneus longus ligamentoplasty for chronic instability of the distal tibiofibular syndesmosis. Foot Ankle Int 2003; 24(5):392–7.

72. Buchhorn T, Sabeti-Aschraf M, Dlaska CE, et al. Combined medial and lateral anatomic ligament reconstruction for chronic rotational instability of the ankle. Foot Ankle Int 2011;32(12):1122–6.

73. Lack W, Phisitkul P, Femino JE. Anatomic deltoid ligament repair with anchor-to-post suture reinforcement: technique tip. Iowa Orthop J 2012;32:227–30.

74. Dodd A, Daniels TR. Total ankle replacement in the presence of talar varus or valgus deformities. Foot Ankle Clin 2017;22(2):277–300.

75. Schuberth JM, Christensen JC, Seidenstricker CL. Total ankle replacement with severe valgus deformity: technique and surgical strategy. J Foot Ankle Surg 2017;56(3):618–27.

76. Pellegrini MJ, Torres N, Cuchacovich NR, et al. Chronic deltoid ligament insufficiency repair with Internal Brace augmentation. Foot Ankle Surg 2019;25(6): 812–8.

Moving?

Make sure your subscription moves with you!

To notify us of your new address, find your **Clinics Account Number** (located on your mailing label above your name), and contact customer service at:

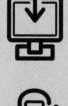

Email: journalscustomerservice-usa@elsevier.com

800-654-2452 (subscribers in the U.S. & Canada)
314-447-8871 (subscribers outside of the U.S. & Canada)

Fax number: 314-447-8029

Elsevier Health Sciences Division
Subscription Customer Service
3251 Riverport Lane
Maryland Heights, MO 63043

*To ensure uninterrupted delivery of your subscription, please notify us at least 4 weeks in advance of move.

ELSEVIER